Practical Magic For The Kitchen Witch

I0449292

Practical Magic For The Kitchen Witch

P. M. Schamel

ISBN : 1-4196-0149-0

To order additional copies, please contact us.
BookSurge, LLC
www.booksurge.com
1-866-308-6235
orders@booksurge.com

Practical Magic For The Kitchen Witch

Table Of Contents

Overview

In this abbreviated history of witchcraft I would like to take a moment to tell you a little bit about myself and what witchcraft means to me. This is my personal view. I am not claming to be an expert on history, but I have done a great deal of study on the subject and as a freethinking individual I have many theories on the matter. I would also like to take this moment to thank you personally for reading. Even if you just pick this book up at random out of curiosity that is a step in the right direction. All answers start with a question and knowledge comes out of the need for answers.

What does it mean to be a Witch? Well if you asked 20 people that question you would probably get 20 different answers. Some say it is the oldest known religion while others say it is just a different way of life; for me being a Witch means being responsible for my own choices. I am the one to choose my destiny instead of just riding along on someone else's grand adventure. It takes discipline and nurturing to learn what I really want and need to know, and I am awed by the opportunity. For me witchcraft is a way of expressing myself and forming a balance that I have been missing in my life. There are many different practices within the realm of paganism but no single practice fits me exactly. I am an eclectic. I have molded bits and pieces of the various different beliefs to my own way of thinking, to make it personal. I know that some would disagree with that, but for me it works.

I am not only Pagan, I am a Witch, but not in the way you might think. I don't have green skin or a pointy hat or a wart on the tip of my nose. Even if I did I would use magic to get rid of it. I do have a black cat, though, that sits at my feet whenever I cast a spell. Yes, I cast spells, make potions, and brew teas, but I don't follow any one set of beliefs. I don't worship gods or goddesses although I do believe in them and respect them. I just don't see them as a separate part of us, any more than I see my hand as a separate part of my body. Instead, I have faith that all things are connected in all ways. This applies to the physical as well as the metaphysical. Just because I can't see it does not mean it's not there. Most of all, I feel that we are all responsible for our own actions. Everything affects everything else.

I am not a high priestess nor do I agree with any hierarchy within Witchcraft or Paganism. Though that choice is right for some, it isn't right for me. I simply believe that there are some people who have studied longer and know more than I do. That does not make them my leaders, just my really smart friends. I would never dream of telling others how they should believe. I would only encourage them to expand on their shared experiences. If I were to tell you anything at all about how to be a witch, I would say if it works for you and it harms none then go where it leads you. One of the best analogies that I have heard was from a guy that was trying to sell me a vacuum cleaner. He said, "If you can imagine it you should think about it. Once you have thought it over, if your common sense still says you can, then, yeah you can probably do that".

For me, being a Witch means I can do what I inherently know is right without the pretences of creating a better after-life. After all, if I spend all of my time worrying about what happens after I die, I will have missed the point of living. I believe we are here to learn from and to care for all life, so that once we have left this area of existence we may become a different part of the continuing energy that makes up all things.

Of course, my choice did not go over well with my very Christian family. To tell the truth they still don't agree, but that's okay. I never asked them or anyone else to agree with it. The point is that it is *my* choice to make. That is the one thing that I think everyone faced with this decision should know. It is okay to follow your own path. Even if the people around you disagree, in the end it is *your* life to live. If you feel compelled to walk down that road, you will never find happiness until you do. Just know that you are not alone in your decision. You will meet many different kinds of people who all have something to share. If you keep an open mind you can learn a lot about yourself and your place in the world around you. It was tough for me in the beginning, but I have endured and become stronger for it. Along the way I have met some very interesting people, not all of them good, not all of them bad, but each of them a wonderful experience and opportunity to learn from. Some of those lessons I did not realize until much later in my life, but as I look back I can see how important it was for me to have that experience even if I didn't understand why until now.

I was thirteen when I started seeking a new faith. I remember asking my mother, *"How old does a child have to be before they are able to choose their own religion?"* She told me then, *"When the child has studied enough to understand what that religion is all about and when it feels right, then it is time for the child to choose."* I was fifteen when I began to practice witchcraft and I learned very quickly that this was *not* what my mother had in mind when I told her I wanted to convert. So, I had to hide what I was doing from my family. I held my solitary rituals out behind the garage and cast spells while no one was around. I maintained this secret life for a long time. It wasn't fun, in fact it was very lonely to know that I had found this wonderful thing that made me feel happy and balanced and to know that I couldn't share it with the people in my life that I loved the most. I found some comfort and a lot of knowledge (no matter how misguided) in my friends but it wasn't the same as being able to share it with family, someone who would help me to grow and nurture my interests and gifts. My mother found out I was studying witchcraft when I was seventeen. I tried to explain it to her, but she still didn't accept the fact that *this* was my choice. She tried a number of things to "save me". She banned me from seeing my friends and she forced me to attend her church. I was even sent to a psychologist to confirm that I had a "problem". He agreed that I did have an issue with conformity (something I feel is of key importance to anyone who chooses his or her own path), but he also had to admit that I was not a threat to myself or anyone else. Unsatisfied with that result, she then took me to see a Catholic priest (even though she was a Baptist at that time). The priest did not believe in Witchcraft either. According to him I had a wonderful imagination and an insatiable curiosity. My mother then tried to enroll me in a Christian school. I guess they did not like the answers I gave at the interview, because they declined my application.

Though I have a great deal of respect for other religions and I understand that my mother was only reacting to something that she didn't understand, I began to resent the implications that I was not capable of making this kind of decision for myself. I had researched many aspects of religion before I made my choice, something that I highly encourage others to do regardless of what religion if any they choose. Knowledge is one of the greatest forms of power and something we all have access to. After the psychologist, the priest and the rejection letter from the Christian school, I began to fully understand how the Witches in Europe and the American colonies must have felt during the Inquisition and the infamous Salem Witch Trials.

We have all heard the story as it was beautifully depicted in the movie and play, "The Crucible" by Arthur Miller, who oddly enough went through a similar ordeal 3 years after writing the play. He was called to testify at the McCarthy anti-communist hearings and was held in contempt for his refusal to release the names of people he purportedly saw at a Communist writer's meeting. It still saddens me to think about what so many innocent people have gone through and I am angry that people are still being condemned over 300 years after the Salem trials. It just goes to show how much ignorance and fear can affect the world we live in and how extremely important knowledge truly is to everyone.

Almost 1000 years ago in 1012 A.D., the Catholic Church ruled that heresy was punishable by imprisonment and death. The term "heresy" was, and still is defined as "any belief at variance with established beliefs, customs etc". Basically, if your government believes in one thing and you believe in another or the same thing only differently, that is heresy and that makes you the heretic. In 1230 A.D. the Inquisitions started in Europe, and by the late 1500's and early 1600's it was not safe to believe in a different manner than what the government told you to believe. The church and the king feared what they could not control. To them, anyone who could manipulate the very forces of nature had to be extremely powerful and that scared them. The practice of Christianity dictated that only "God" could manipulate the natural forces. If the common person, or pagan, could learn to do this it would directly affect the power the church held over them. The Church depended upon the ignorance and fear of its followers to maintain its authority. They had to find a way to regain control over this group of people who seemed to have slipped away from their grasp. It wasn't illegal to be a Witch, (the church and government had no official position on that yet), but to be a "heretic" was against the law. Since witchcraft (the act of manipulating the forces nature) was not illegal, but it was the basis for this potential loss of control, the officials had to devise a way to legally put an end to witchcraft. The only way they could put anyone on trial for witchcraft was if they could prove heresy was involved. This became the loophole that gave way to the death of witchcraft and its practitioners. Thus, sanctioned by the church and the king, anything that could not be explained became suspect of heresy.

By the mid 1600's to early 1700's this heresy craze had swept into the American colonies. In Salem, MA in 1692 A.D. the infamous Salem Witch trials began. They lasted for almost a year before anyone stepped in. This was not to put an end to the madness, but rather to change the rules by which someone could be tried for witchcraft. Witches could still be put on trial, but there were new limits on the amount of torture the jury could inflict to get a confession and they now had to supply at least a little evidence for a conviction. A lot of people died during that time and the ones who survived had to hide what they were doing or else risk being imprisoned and/or killed.

Even if the accused didn't consider the rituals by which they lived their lives to be witchcraft, someone else's perception could now get them killed. In a way, those who hated and feared the concept of "witchcraft" made witchcraft real. So what happened to this form of witchcraft?

We know very little about what happened to witchcraft prior to its rebirth in 1939 by Gerald B. Gardner. Unfortunately most of what was written about it was either destroyed in the panic or completely biased. There is no evidence that witchcraft in any form survived the trials of long ago. I believe however that some of the men and women who practiced what was considered to be witchcraft, or natural magic, must have found a new way to continue their practices while not raising the suspicions of their friends, families and neighbors. It is my theory that they transformed their craft into something more practical. I suspect that it was moved indoors and became what we now know as Kitchen Witchery. They probably took everyday utensils and charged them with their magic intent in order to continue the work that was needed. The cooking spoon replaced the wand, the pot replaced the cauldron, and the herbs and other magical ingredients were added with care to every carefully planned meal. Some of these magical recipes have endured over time. Why else would we still serve black-eyed peas on New Years Day? I believe magic must have adapted or we wouldn't have the version of it that we practice today. The best I can tell, and this is just my speculation, is that it changed and thus endured. The practice of witchcraft became so subtle that it passed through the burning times undetected until it was safe once again to practice it out in the open. Of course by that time the world was a different place. What emerged was a new version of the old ways.

Let me say here that there are a lot of people who try to claim to be born Witches. I do not believe there is any such heredity. By saying to be a "true Witch" you must have ancestors who were witches is like saying to be a "true Christian" you must have ancestors who were Christian. Being Pagan or Wiccan or a Witch of any kind is a choice in how you live your life just as it is for being a Christian. You do not have to be Pagan to be a Witch; it just happens that most of us are due to the general lack of acceptance among most Christian faiths. This is not to down-play the importance of tradition. Magic is deeply rooted in traditions. Even my mother still practices some of the oldest known traditions. Of course she refuses to accept that they are Pagan, but she still decorates an evergreen tree and hangs a wreath of evergreen and holly on her door every year. She also sets out carved pumpkins, and dyes eggs with bright colors even if she doesn't know why or what these traditional symbols of the holidays mean. These Pagan practices are an important part of our lives, even if no one remembers where they started or why we do them. It is proof that magic is still alive and the practice of witchcraft never truly died out. Magic and witchcraft have evolved and hopefully so have we. This doesn't make it any better or any worse than what it once was; magic simply *is* and it is in everything. Don't believe me? Give a bouquet of flowers or bake some cookies for someone when they are feeling down, see if their faces don't light up and just like magic they feel better, and so do you.

Today, Kitchen Witchery is just as powerful as it has always been. Whether it is a plate of cookies after a hard day or chicken soup when someone is sick there has always been a little magic brewing in the kitchen. Even non-witches have to admit that some of the best moments in their lives have been spent either in someone's kitchen or enjoying the meals that were prepared in one. Food, after all, connects everything. It is one of the basic elements of life. Nothing symbolizes the importance of food more that the simple act of praying over it and giving thanks for it.

It is not just good food that comes out of kitchens either. There are plenty of medicines found in the cupboards of almost every kitchen as well. Just take a look in yours. I am willing to bet you will find you already have a majority of the ingredients needed to combat some of today's more common ailments. When I first started collecting herbs for my craft I was amazed to find most of them in my own spice rack right next to the stove. These are things that I used on a daily basis without thinking about what applications they have to magic. If my son got a cold or my husband banged his thumb, I had the means to help them right at my fingertips; it was just a matter of learning how to use it. Maybe it is because the kitchen is home to so many wonderful things that it is associated with the feelings of warmth, safety and comfort. After all it is the one place in the house where all five of the elements (earth, air, fire, water and you) can be found just about any time.

Today we are lucky to be able to practice our crafts out in the open. Don't get me wrong, we are still persecuted; we are judged and mocked and other people don't always treat us very kindly, but at least it is no longer legal to burn us at the stake. We can proudly wave our wands and brooms, we can even hold our rituals out in the open air; but there is something deep inside that still holds a special appreciation for good old fashion kitchen magic. Cooking and stirring, boiling and baking, and communing with one another, now that is powerful magic! It kind of reminds me of the fabled old witches who were always adding eyes of newts and tongues of frogs to boiling cauldrons. One has to wonder what they were really brewing. Were they cooking up some kind of potion or just making dinner? It is possible they were doing both.

As the burning times reached their peak, people could be killed for simply growing the wrong things in their garden. In order for the witches to be able to grow what they needed they had to change a few of the names. Some of those odd ingredients we hear in old spells as they are being cast into the cauldron are just everyday common herbs and flowers. Bloody fingers and ram's heads are actually foxglove and valerian root; you didn't think we would really put a whole ram's head in a pot now did you? It would never have fit. The names given to the different plants helped to shroud magic in a cloak of mystery. They are fun to play with and interesting to know, but not important for the spell to work. If you want to freak out your friends as your cooking just spout off a few obscure ingredients as you go. Since most of the plants where named for what they resembled it wouldn't be difficult to figure out what they are. You could do some research as a fun hobby. The odd names served another purpose as well. They made the rhymes easier to remember. It was too dangerous to have a written account of the spells and their ingredients so little poems or rhymes were created to help remember them and to make it possible to pass them on without being detected. In this same way some of the oldest nursery rhymes told of historical events, such as the fall of London Bridge or the Black Plague. Today's magic works much the same way. Though the spells do not have to rhyme exactly and you by no means have to be a great poet to write spells, the rhymes add rhythm and music to your work as well as adding a little flair. Use your imagination, a rhyme thesaurus or ask the muses for some help to make the magic your own. Magic should be personal, just so long as it is clear what you are asking for. It is a natural part of the world we live in. Just as you would tend to your garden to help it grow, so should you tend to your magic. Nurture it, and cultivate its powers, and watch as it grows stronger and more beautiful with each new season.

By the magic of these flowers
Rosemary, Ash and Rue
I sow with love, the seeds of power
To make all my dreams come true.
Blessed Be

I would like to give a special thank you to my husband and my son. I know it has been rough going these last few months but thank you for your love and support. With all of my heart this book is written for you guys. Pat and Emory, I love you both.

PART 1

A word of warning

There is a certain amount of freedom that comes from creating concoctions. I love cooking and brewing the special recipes and knowing that it is not just a matter of throwing some stuff in a pot but a conscious act of love and magic. But with that freedom comes a great deal of responsibility. There are a great many things that if not used wisely can cause injury or even death. I have found that herbal healing is not for the careless or for people who are not willing to devote a great deal of dedication and discipline to the craft. As with all magic it must be used responsibly. In my practice I focus on intent and energy, but not the specific deities, planets or elements that some may choose to invoke. You may of course apply these things to the gods or goddesses of your choice. I do adhere to the basic rule of witchcraft. There are also simple guidelines that are important for budding new Witches to learn, and for seasoned Witches it never hurts to brush up.

One of the best things about magic is that we are limited in its use only by our imaginations. We have but one basic rule to follow in order for our workings to turn out the way we want, which is *"Harm none"*. That's it, Our one rule. We do have a few guidelines, just common sense and good manners really, one of which is *"Do not manipulate the will of others"*. Free will is very important to magic. I am not saying it is impossible to make someone do as you wish, I am just saying it is a bad idea. It is always best to have permission, even if your intention is of the best of heart. This leads us to another good point when dealing with magic, *"what you send out you shall receive three fold"*. So it is best if you only send out good energy, after all there is enough negative energy in the world today without drawing in more.

Magic can be very simple and basic or it can be very complex. In my experience it works just as well either way. You do not need elaborate dress or eloquent wording to get your intent out there. Even though sometimes dressing up and making it formal can be fun, it is not always practical. I would like to concentrate mainly on simple everyday magic here. The kind of thing you can work into your everyday life. You can add these things to your daily cooking or routine without much more effort than boiling some water. When stating your desire, speak clearly and be careful of what you ask for. You will get it even if it is not the way you thought it would be.

There are many paths to healing and many things both common and obscure that can be used. In this book I will concentrate mainly on the healing powers of herbs and plants that you may find commonly around your house. Some of the items listed here can be found in your cupboards while others may grow wild or in your garden. Still others you may need to search for at your local occult shop or at a nursery. Just keep a watchful eye out and you may find that quite a few of the ingredients are not as elusive as you once thought. I once found the ingredients for a money spell in a store brand tea bag. So you just never know where they might turn up.

Also, though we are dealing with the medicinal use of herbs I do not mean to imply that anything in this book should take the place of medical advice. The use of herbs and diet should always be discussed with your doctor. This is simply a guide to alternatives. I have never personally been a big fan of drugs if I can find a more natural way to fix the problem, but there are some things that really do require medication prescribed by a doctor. I take comfort in knowing that in some cases science has found a safe way that was at least inspired by nature, to treat the illness. Some doctors are willing to work with you on your choice for natural and safe herbal alternatives. Tell your doctor if you are taking any herbs, and always check for drug interactions.

Herbs and pregnancy

Some herbs should not be used or handled by women who are pregnant, nursing, or of childbearing age. Please use caution before using or handling herbs under these circumstances.

Poisonous and Sensitive

All plants should be handled and or used with care and caution.

Below is a list of possible reactions to some of the specific plants and herbs. Please read carefully. Not all of the plants listed below are used in the recipes that follow and not all are poisonous or deadly but they may cause undesirable reactions or complications. Please use caution before using these or any plants and herbs. Before using any remedy for the first time, test a small amount and check for any reaction. Some people may have unknown allergies to plants and herbs that they may not be familiar with. Some allergies can build up over time with prolonged use. Every plant and herb may not be listed here, but just because it is not listed as having possible dangers, does not mean you should assume it is safe. If you experience any unusual symptoms or reactions, discontinue use immediately and consult a doctor. Be sure to tell him/her what you have taken, how it was prepared and how much at which times.

Alfalfa—Do not use Alfalfa sprout if you have a family history of Lupus.

Allspice—May cause inflammation to people with sensitive skin or eczema. The concentrated oil should not be swallowed; 1 teaspoon may cause nausea, vomiting and convulsions.

Aloe Vera—(dried juice) strong laxative

Angelica—uterine stimulant, should not be taken by persons with tendencies toward diabetes as it increases the sugar in urine.

Bayberry—Do not use for children under 2 years. For older children or people over age 65 start with low doses and increase as needed. Large doses may cause stomach distress. Bayberry changes the way the body uses sodium and potassium. Not for use while pregnant or nursing.

Belladonna—(*also known as Deadly Nightshade*) all parts, especially the unripe berries, are fatal causing digestive disturbance and problems with the nervous system.

Calamus—uterine stimulant should be avoided during pregnancy

Caraway—Is a central nervous system stimulant. Prolonged use can lead to potential kidney damage.

Castor Bean—the seeds are fatal. Death has occurred by ingesting even one or two.

Chamomile—People who have allergies to ragweed may have an allergic reaction to chamomile. Use small doses to determine effect.

Cinnamon—skin irritant, circulatory stimulant repeated use may cause allergic reactions.

Clove—may cause skin irritation, avoid while pregnant.

Comfrey—Use of comfrey has been associated with liver damage.

Dong Quai—can act as a stimulant on the central nervous system and as a uterine stimulant. It is not recommended in large doses during pregnancy, excessive menstrual flow, or while taking blood thinners. People with fair skin may become photosensitive.

Eucalyptus—should not allow fumes around infants. It can cause difficulty in breathing.

Evening primrose oil—should be taken with food to minimize gastric distress, also take with vitamin E. Not for use while pregnant or nursing or while on anti-psychotic medication. Do not use with schizophrenia or epilepsy. EPO promotes estrogen production and therefore should not be taken by women with estrogen related breast cancers.

Feverfew—should not be used by pregnant women due to uterine stimulation. It may cause ulcers in the mouth if chewed.

Ginger—is a profound and immediate stimulant.

Ginkgo—Do not use with blood thinners, aspirin or high doses of vitamin E

Goldenseal—anti-convulsive effect on uterus

Hemlock—is fatal and resembles large wild carrots.

Hops—should not be used in cases of severe depression.

Hyssop—the oil may cause seizures, avoid if pregnant with high blood pressure or epilepsy.

Juniper—should not be used if you have kidney disease or during pregnancy.

Kava—is a mild narcotic. High doses can lead to muscle weakness, dizziness or liver damage. Do not consume alcohol, drive or use where quick reflexes are required. Do not use while pregnant, nursing or being treated for depression. Kava has been associated with liver damage if over-used.

Licorice—may affect electrolyte balance with extended use of large amounts, can raise blood pressure and cause retention of sodium Do not use with hypertension, kidney disease or during pregnancy. Do not combine with diuretics.

Lobelia—is a powerful respiratory stimulant.

Mandrake—poisonous

May apple—contains at least 16 known toxic principles mostly in the roots. Though children have often eaten the apples with out any effect, too much may cause diarrhea.

Mistletoe—berries are fatal if eaten.

Passion flower—has a depressive effect on the central nervous system.

Oak—foliage and acorns affect the kidneys; symptoms appear gradually over several days or weeks when taken in large amounts

Rosemary—circulatory and nervous system stimulant, should not be handled while pregnant. May irritate stomach, intestines and kidneys if over-used internally. Avoid using with high blood pressure.

St. John' Wort—Constant or over-use can lead to photosensitivity.

Tea tree—may cause skin irritation

White sage—Use only as a weak tea, ingesting too much can cause convulsions.

White willow—contains aspirin. Do not use if allergic or sensitive to aspirin.

Wild/cultivated cherry—twigs and foliage contains a compound that releases cyanide when eaten.

Yarrow—lowers blood pressure.

PART 2

Before you start

Working with herbs and plants grown in your own garden is best. That way you can be sure of how they were grown and processed. You know what kind of soil was used and what they have been exposed to. It is best if you do not use any chemical insecticides or fertilizers if you can keep from it. While sowing, growing, and cultivating your herbs it helps if you can form a bonding relationship with them. I know that may sound strange, but all living things need love and attention. As you water and tend to your garden speak softly to the plants. Encouraging them to grow and caressing them gently will make for a more positive experience for both you and your plants.

If you cannot grow your herbs or plants or just choose to use the store-bought ones you have in your kitchen, it will not change the outcome of your recipes. You will need to use a little more preparation though. Arrange your herbs in a neat and easy to access manner. Spend a few minutes with each one and get to know it personally. Become familiar with each individual flavor, smell, and appearance as well as the way those flavors and aromas react to each other. Some herbs form a synergistic relationship to others to create a unique blending. Also, some herbs are stronger than others and can easily overpower your recipe. With a little practice, you will learn how to use them in balance and harmony with one another for your desired purpose.

Before starting any work, it helps to have a well-cleaned, organized area to work in. Aside from the necessary day-to-day cleaning you may want to go through your kitchen with a smoldering bundle of white sage to clear it of all negative energy. If you do not have sage, a little salt water sprinkled about, or any other cleansing ritual will work just as well. Using a broom (a corn broom or one you have made specifically for rituals is best but your house broom will be fine), sweep clear all negative energy. You should do this each time you work. It is always nice to keep the energy positive and happy. You may want to play your favorite music, burn some incense or a nice scented candle, whatever it is that makes you feel good. Visualize your space as being protected and cleared of all negative energy.

If you feel the need you may also cleanse the tools of your craft by carefully washing each instrument pots, pans, spoons, jars etc. You can wash them in running water or let them soak for a while in salt water. Allow them to dry in the sun for the magical energy it provides. The waxing moonlight works well for empowering tools as well. There are also several herbs that can be used to cleanse your tools, such as benzoin and clove. Frankincense and myrrh can be used for consecration as well. Personally I feel that the magic of the kitchen, as well as the tools and the recipes are inherently pure and loving. This makes the cleansing of the pots and pans redundant for me, unless the day has been particularly stressful, or my husband and I have recently had an argument in the kitchen. Then I may clean the instruments just to help re-center everything. It never hurts to be cautious just in case.

When you are ready to begin preparing your remedy, gather all of your ingredients together. Taking each one in hand, bless and charge them for your use. Each herb contains inherent properties that can be brought out by concentrating your magic and intent. Since some herbs have more than one property, charge only what you will need for each use. Keep the thought of your purpose firmly in your mind. If it is to heal, think of the person and visualize them as being healthy, see them wrapped in a green glow and picture the ailment being forced out. If it is love then picture that. Visualize all of the things that remind you of love or make you feel loved. It takes a lot of energy and concentration but you will get the hang of it quickly, and you will begin to feel a bit of yourself being connected with everything else as you work. When you have finished ensure that you bless the final product and give an offering of thanks and gratitude to the plants, herbs, and flowers as well as to the powers that be for their aid in your purpose. Clean up the area as a sign of respect for yourself and your space. Offer any unused ingredients back to the earth or begin a compost pile for herbal fertilizers. Giving back to the land and the energy that has aided you is one way to ensure that it stays balanced and happy.

Preparing herbal remedies

Herbs, berries, flowers and other parts of the plants can be used in one or more of the different methods. Some parts of the plants cannot be used at all, it is important to know when which part is used. It is also important to note that some remedies can take some time to prepare. In that case you will want to make them in advance. For instance, when the frost is starting to lift and the days are beginning to get warmer, you know that bug bites are just around the corner. Basil tinctures are great for itchy bug bites but they take 2 weeks to prepare. By making the tincture in advance you will be ready and it keeps for up to 2 years in a dark bottle. Other remedies should not be made more than 24 hours in advance. Knowing which is which can save time and money as well as stress.

When it comes to preparing herbal remedies the less stress there is the better it will be. Remember try to keep the energy as positive as you can. Have fun with it and try different experiments. A number of these herbs and plants can just be charged and added to every day meals for a magical boost and a new unique flavor. I taught my husband (the chef) to put fennel in tomato sauce when he had trouble with a fungal infection.

He loved the new taste enough to try it in more recipes, and I am happy to say the fungus didn't like it so much. For some remedies the method used is a matter of preference, while for others the method is important for the proper result. The majority of the following recipes will be recommended in teas. For some recipes the use of other methods of preparation will be required either alone or in combination with one another. It is important to know how to prepare each.

How to make...

(All methods are in alphabetical order)

Broths: Broths and teas are used much the same way and are prepared in almost the same manner. The main difference being that instead of using just water as the base of a broth you will use bouillon cubes or an actual soup mixture. This helps some of the spicier or more pungent herbs go down a little easier. For example you can make a tea using basil or cayenne, but the taste or hotness may leave a little to be desired, so a broth may be useful in masking some harsh or spicy flavors.

Capsules: Use dry, powdered herbs to place inside an empty capsule. This is useful for particularly bitter or fowl tasting herbs such as valerian. You will need to use a mortar and pestle for this or lacking this tool, a bean grinder will work just as well. Some herbs, roots and seeds take quite a bit of effort to reduce to a powder but in the end you will feel much more satisfied with the outcome.

Compress: Soak a piece of cloth in a hot decoction of the herb(s) you are using. Wring out excess liquid and place on the affected area. Repeat as needed each time the cloth becomes cool. You may add tinctures and essential oils to the liquid as well.

Cream: In a double boiler melt two ounces of beeswax. Add one cup of carrier oil, (olive, vegetable etc.) and blend. Add Two ounces of desired herb(s). Simmer for about 20 minutes while mixing well. Add one or two drops of Benzoin tincture as a preservative and strain through cheesecloth into a sterilized jar.

Decoctions: Place one to two teaspoons of herb(s) in one cup of cold water. Bring to a boil. Keep covered and simmer for about 10 minutes. The usual dosage will be one cup three times a day unless otherwise noted. You should not prepare decoctions more than 24 hours ahead of use.

Infusions: Add one to two teaspoons of dried (or two to four teaspoons fresh) herb(s) to one cup boiling water. Let it set for 10 minutes. The usual dosage is one cup three times a day, hot or cold, unless otherwise indicated. It should not be prepared more than 24 hours before use. (Infusions for colds and flu are almost always taken hot).

Inhalants/steam: Add decoction, two teaspoons of tincture or one or two drops of oils, to boiling water. Use the steam for skin problems or as inhalant for breathing or sinus trouble.

Lozenges: Use about 4 ounces of the herbal decoction of your choice. In a bowl mix herb(s) with enough powdered marshmallow root to form a thick paste. Add 3-4 drops of peppermint oil. Pinch off small pieces and shape. Place on wax paper and allow drying for several hours. Store covered in the refrigerator and use to soothe sore or irritated throats.

Oils: Place a jar filled with the intended herb(s) in a saucepan of water. Cover herb(s) with oil (olive, vegetable etc.) Bring water to a medium temperature and simmer for three hours. Strain the oil through cheesecloth. Repeat the process using the same oil and fresh herb(s) to make oil stronger. Keep oil in a dark colored bottle.

Ointments: Ointments will not absorb into the skin as easily as creams will but are used topically for different treatments. To make an ointment place the herbs you wish to use in a double boiler and melt enough petroleum jelly to cover the herb(s). Simmer until the herb(s) are crisp. Strain into a jar while hot and let cool.

Poultice: Mix chopped herb(s) or powdered seeds with boiling water and make a pulp. Place pulp in cheesecloth and apply to affected area while hot. Leave on until it cools then replace.

Syrups: Add 1 ¾ cup brown sugar or a honey and sugar mix to two cups infusion or decoction. Heat the mixture until the sugar dissolves then pour it into a clean glass bottle. Store it in the refrigerator. Use one teaspoon three times a day.

Tea: Place one to two teaspoons of dried herbs or three to four teaspoons of fresh herbs in a mesh tea strainer or tea bag. Steep the herbs in one cup of hot water for three to five minutes unless otherwise specified.

Tincture: Place four ounces of dried herb(s) in a glass jar and add two cups of vodka. Place the lid on the jar tightly and leave for two weeks, shaking occasionally. Strain through cheesecloth into a dark glass bottle. Keep closed tightly for up to two years. Use 15 drops three times a day unless otherwise noted.

PART 3

Magical recipes and remedies

Addiction

Addiction is one of the hardest things to deal with in our live. We may become addicted to just about anything that supplies up with gratification. Work, sex, chocolate, even the internet all have the potential to become addictive. The key is to try and balance these things with the rest of our lives. If you feel you or a loved one may be forming an addiction it is important to address the issue as soon as possible. Try to set limit as to how long you or they can participate in that activity during one setting. Two of the more dangerous forms of addiction, smoking and alcoholism are listed in this section. The remedies below can also be applied with other remedies such as those for stress to combat these and most any addictions.

Alcoholism

Alcoholism is a serious and potentially fatal disease. It affects millions of people every year. These remedies will not cure an alcoholic, but they will help with the symptoms of alcoholism. Use of these remedies in cooperation with love and support from friends and family members, as well as other remedies, to combat symptoms such as depression, fatigue, and anxiety will greatly increase the chances of recovery.

Angelica: The regular use of Angelica root can lessen the cravings for alcohol by creating distaste for alcoholic beverages. The root can be dried and ground into a powder for capsules or used as an infusion for teas. It can also be baked like a potato and eaten as a sweet treat.

Evening primrose oil: The oil comes from the seeds of the primrose flower, which blooms at night and is used to reduce the symptoms of alcohol withdrawal. It is also beneficial for healing cirrhosis of the liver. The leaves are tasty in a salad.

Hops: The flower may be uses as a tea to decrease the desire for alcohol. It also aids in toning the liver. Hops flower is a powerful depressant and should not be used with those having problems with depression. Passion flower is milder, but either should be used regularly.

Milk Thistle: The seeds can help protect the liver from damage due to alcohol by regenerating the liver cells. The seeds are used in capsules or can be ground and used as a coffee substitute.

Mullein: The tea can be drunk as a liver tonic.

<u>Stop smoking</u>

Dropping the smoking habit is not easy. Non-smokers have no idea how hard it can be. Even if you want to kick the habit, sometimes the stress and anxiety of everyday life can just be too much. Then you add the stress of withdrawals and you have a really bad day ahead of you. This is a small section but if used in combination with other sections to reduce the symptoms associated with quitting, it can make a big difference in your chances for success.

Calamus: The stems or bits of dried roots can be chewed.

Licorice: Pieces of the dried root can be chewed to reduce withdrawal.

Red clover: The tea from this sweet flower can help to kick the habit.

Blood

Our blood is the basic unit of life. It touches every part of our body so it is good to keep it in balance. The foods below are used to clean, purify, detoxify and generally keep our blood healthy. Some of these remedies are focused on specific blood aliments while others are good for keeping the blood healthy in general.

Alfalfa: When you eat alfalfa as part of a good diet it acts as a mild blood thinner. The health benefits that come from adding a few sprouts to some of your favorite healthy foods are overwhelming.

American Ginseng: When compared to its Asian cousins, American Ginseng supplies a milder version of the same effect. Used in teas or taken as capsules the Ginseng family works to lower blood pressure and help regulate blood sugar.

Apple cider vinegar: Dinking a few tablespoons of apple cider vinegar daily helps to lower blood pressure. It thins the blood enough to allow it to flow freely but it also help the blood to clot, which can be useful for people who suffer from ailments such as hemophilia. It also helps to oxidize the blood. You might try replacing your caffeine rich teas and coffees with a glass or two of apple cider vinegar and water.

Basil: The use of basil in teas and cooking can help to lower blood pressure. It is just one of its many benefits.

Bladderwrack: A member of the kelp family works to purify the blood when eaten. Kelp is high in dietary fiber and calcium and low in cholesterol, which makes it a healthy choice for salads and sandwiches. Bladderwrack or Kelp can be found in most fish markets.

Cayenne: Adding a little spice to your food can help in more ways than one. When added to food cayenne works in the body to clean the bloodstream as well as increase metabolism and produce sweating.

Celery: Adding celery seeds to foods such as pasta sauces, soups and salads can not only bring a new flavor to your meal but also help to lower cholesterol and fight high blood pressure.

Dong quai: Also known as Chinese Angelica, a greenish white flower, is not to be confused with the common Angelica plant. The root extract of Dong quai can be used by men and women as a blood purifying tonic though its primary use is to regulate the female menstrual cycle.

Echinacea: This is another herb with multiple benefits. Taking Echinacea can not only lessen your chances of getting sick and speed up your recovery time, but it is also used in teas to purify the blood.

Garlic: When added to food or taken daily in capsules Garlic helps to lower blood cholesterol and aid in blood flow. It is a mild blood thinner. Not just for Italian foods anymore, Garlic can be added to almost anything. Try it in eggs with some of your favorite fresh veggies or cooked with chicken.

Linden: The lovely little linden flower can help to lower your blood pressure. It may be used with Hawthorn, *Yarrow and *European Mistletoe in teas and decoctions.

Olive: The olive leaf extract fights high blood pressure and increases blood flow. It also makes a great tasting and healthy salad dressing. Try olive oil as cooking oil in place of lard or grease.

Salad dressing

Mix Olive leaf extract with apple cider vinegar, crushed garlic, crushed red pepper or cayenne and a pinch of salt, shake well before each use.

Passion Flower: The pretty purple flower contains a powerful sedative that has been used safely on adults and children. Among its many uses Passion flower can be used to lower blood pressure.

Rose: Rose hips can be used to help heal and prevent the rupture of small blood vessels. It also strengthens the heart.

White Willow: The bark of the willow tree can be used as an anticoagulant. Much like aspirin, the bark is used to prevent heart attack and stroke.

Yerba Mate: Use in teas to reduce blood pressure. It is a great pick me up without Ephedra.

To lower blood sugar

1 part bean pods
1 part nettle leaves
2 parts birch leaves
6 parts bilberry leaves
Steep 1 tablespoon of mixture in ½ cup boiling water
Take ½ cup 3 times daily.

<u>To increase sugar tolerance</u>

Pumpkin seeds (peeled)
Valerian root
Bilberry leaves
Mix equal parts and steep 1 tablespoon in 1 cup of boiling
water. Take 1 cup in mouthful doses, unsweetened, throughout
the day.

Circulation

Most of the remedies in this section can be used in
conjunction with the remedies for blood. Keeping the blood
cleaned and in good circulation can help in many ways to stop
swelling, coldness and tingling of the limbs.

Bayberry: You know the sweet smelling holiday candles.
They get their wonderful wax right from these berries. While
the wax coating is great for candles the berries may be used as a
poultice to stimulate circulation and tone tissues. Used in a tea
they also promote sweating.

Clove: Clove is a tasty, sweet spice that is often overlooked.
When eaten clove raises body temperature and promotes
sweating. You can use the whole clove or the oil for added
flavor.

Ginger: The same stuff you eat to cleanse the palate when
you eat sushi can help to cleanse the blood stream. Eating
ginger also promotes sweating.

Linden: A beautiful addition to any garden or walkway
Linden can be used as a tea to increase circulation.

Rosemary: Use the oil of the rosemary plant in a massage oil,
liniment, compress or bath to increase circulation. It can also
be added to cooking for a little flavor that goes a long way.

Circulation tea

Calamus
Hawthorn
Shavegrass
Motherwort
Cornsilk
Lemon balm (lemongrass)
Yarrow
Valerian
Olive
Mix into tea and drink 2-3 cups daily

Heart health

Heart conditions are very serious. This is another of those things I would recommend a doctor for. If you are on heart medication, do not attempt to replace your medicine with herbs all at once. Start slow and build up. With healthy diet and exercise and the right heart-building nutrients it is possible that you may free yourself from a medicated life, but this takes time. So relax and be patient.

Angelica: Used as a tincture or a tea, it can help reduce the risk of heart problems. There are many other ways to use Angelica such as salads and candies.

Bilberry: (Also known as European blueberry) can be eaten to strengthen the heart. Add them to your favorite treat or breakfast in the morning. Used in combination with oats, blueberries are a tasty way to start the day off healthy.

Cayenne: Spice up your heart with the one you love. Not only is cayenne good for your heart it is a lust-invoking spice. It can be added to foods in place of black pepper.

Dong quai: The sweet greenish flowers strengthen the heart when taken.

Hawthorne: This is very good for your heart. Hawthorn can be used in a tea or mixed with your favorite recipes.

Lemon balm: A member of the mint family can be made into a tea or steeped for 1 hour in wine and drunk with dinner. Red wine is best for this. It is also used to make Lemon balm vinegar dressing.

Heart syrup

Hawthorn berry
Motherwort
Gingko leaf
Passion flower
Pau d' Arco
Honey
Brandy

Use the infusions or decoctions mixed with honey and brandy to make syrup. Take 1 teaspoon 3 times a day.

Flax seed butter

2/3 cup finely chopped hazelnuts or walnut
½ cup finely ground flaxseed
2 teaspoons flaxseed oil
½ cup honey

Grind nuts and seeds into a find powder, add to honey and flaxseed oil and blend well. Use as a spread of to flavor oatmeal.

Heart lover's coleslaw salad

Chopped cabbage
Shredded carrots
Thinly sliced apples
Raisins
Scallions or wild onion to taste
1 cup light or fat free salad dressing

1 teaspoon lime juice
1 teaspoon lemon juice
2 tablespoons honey
Combine all vegetables in a large bowl. In a small mixing bowl
stir salad dressing, honey, lemon juice and lime juice. Pour over
vegetables and stir until well coated. Serve chilled.

Cancer

Some types of cancer can be prevented while others seem
to strike for no known reason. We know that a healthy diet is
of key importance in cancer prevention and recovery. These
remedies can help with the prevention of some cancers as well
as to help alleviate some symptoms associated with cancer and
cancer treatment.

Alfalfa: When eaten Alfalfa helps in the prevention of
cancer cell reproduction and aids the body in fighting the
disease. It can also help the body recover from treatments.

Carrot: It may not taste the best but the fresh juice of
whole carrots works in the body to help fight the cancer cells.
Also try fresh carrot soup.

Cinnamon: Fresh or ground cinnamon as well as the oil
can be added to foods and beverages and acts as a preventative
measure for most types of cancer.

Green tea: When used in drinks or in pill form the benefits
of Green tea are remarkable. It has shown significant abilities
for preventing various types of cancer and may be just as
beneficial to the treatment.

Saffron: Saffron has many soothing properties. When
eaten saffron can protect the digestive system against cancer.

Colds and congestion

Wither it is a colds or the flu, allergies or sinus infection; there is always something in the air that can cause congestion and discomfort. Before treatment be sure you understand which it is you are treating. Colds generally set in slowly and are accompanied by coughing, sneezing and runny nose. If you have a cold you may experience mild fatigue, chest discomfort and a sore throat but fever and headache are rare. However with the flu the onset is generally very quick and accompanied by fever, body aches, and chills.

Allergies

From the itchy eyes to the sneezing and irritation, allergies can be a bothersome part of life. Short of the first frost of winter there is little one can hope for as a cure for allergies. Some of these remedies help to prevent the allergies from attacking while others help to ease the symptoms associated with allergies and hay fever.

Alfalfa: Just another of the many wonderful health benefits when eaten as part of a healthy diet. Alfalfa may also be taken in capsule form.

Aloe Vera: Juice made from Aloe Vera is a healthy refreshing choice. It works internally to promote a healthy immune system and as a histamine blocker. You can also try it as a tea.

Caraway: Washing your face in water made from this flower can eliminate the dust and pollens that can cause an allergy attack. You can also breathe as a steam inhalant to aid with the symptoms of allergies.

Echinacea: Is a great immune system booster and can make a short stay of any allergy symptoms. Drink in teas, infusion or taken regularly in capsule form helps to prevent allergies and hay fever attacks.

Rose: Rose Hips are high in vitamin C. They can be used in teas or to make jams and marmalades, especially when mixed with oranges and lemons.

Yerba Mate: When used in a tea it helps to boost the immune system as well as working as an antioxidant.

Allergies tea

2 parts Fenugreek
1 part Horehound
½ part Black Cohosh
1/8 part Lobelia
Mix and steep in a tea drink 3 times a day

Hay fever tea

2 parts Elderflower
1 part Ephedra
1 part Eyebright
1 part Goldenseal
Mix together and steep 1 teaspoon per cup boiling water for 10 minutes.
Drink 1 cup 3 times daily

Bronchitis

When breathing is labored by bronchitis, asthma and other respiratory aliments nothing else seems to matter. This can turn into a serious condition that more than likely will require you to see a doctor. For acute or mild cases as well as to get through the congestion and get the air circulating again try these remedies.

Angelica: Make an infusion by pouring 1 pint of boiling water over 1 ounce of bruised Angelica root (or powdered root). This may be taken several times a day. You can also apply fresh crushed leaves as a poultice to chest and lungs to ease breathing.

Anise: May be used as a tea or to flavor cough syrups. It has a sweat licorice candy taste that is easier for some people to swallow. You can also use Anise as a steam inhalant to help alleviate chest constriction.

Apple cider vinegar: Take one tablespoon of apple cider vinegar in a glass of water. Sip for ½ an hour. Wait ½ hour then repeat. This treatment will relieve the wheezing labored breathing of an asthma attack and may be repeated as often as is necessary until breathing loosens.

Bayberry: When mixed in a tea Bayberry helps increase the circulatory system. It also opens and relaxes the bronchial tubes and helps to break up the mucus.

Benzoin: The tincture made from the gum of the Benzoin tree can be placed on a vaporizer to ease croupy coughs. It can also be used to make cough syrups for bronchitis to help expel mucus.

Eucalyptus: Can be used in capsules or an infusion to relieve bronchitis symptoms. The essential oils used with carrier oil can be used as a rub for the chest or sinus.

Fennel: May be used similar to aniseed. It can be used to flavor cough syrups or teas.

Flax seed: Can be used to make a poultice for chronic coughs.

Garlic: This is probably one of the least expensive and most beneficial treatments for almost anything. 1 clove of garlic eaten raw or crushed and placed in capsules 3 times a day can fight off many forms of infection as well as promote overall good health. The oil in garlic can aid in opening bronchial tubes and lungs when taken orally (40-100 drops per dose).

Lobelia: For use with asthma combine Lobelia with Cayenne, Grindelia, Pill-bearing Surge, Sundew and *Ephedra

Mullein: Use 1-2 teaspoon of the dried leaves in a tea to treat respiratory ailments and relieve pain and spasms. If used in tinctures take ½—1 teaspoon up to 3 times a day. Mullein tastes bitter so you may want to mix it with something or add honey to mask the taste.

Thyme: When used in a steam or taken internally Thyme can help break up the phlegm and congestion caused by bronchitis and other respiratory ailments. Though the active ingredient in thyme is derived from the oils in the leaves Thyme essential oils should not be taken internally. Use the pungent mint flavor leaves to make tea or broth.

Bronchial asthma tea

Sundew
Thyme
Fennel
Silver weed
1 teaspoon of mixture steeped in ½ cup boiling water
Take ½-1 cup daily in mouthful doses, sweetened with honey

Bronchitis tea

Anise
Licorice root
Lance-leaf plantain leaves
Fennel seed

Coltsfoot leaves
1 teaspoon in ½ cup water, bring to a boil
Sweeten with honey or brown sugar
Take ½ cup 3 times daily as hot as possible.

Cold/flu/congestion (sinus)

The high cost of over-the-counter cough and congestion remedies just seem to make a bought of cold or flu feel even worse, especially when they don't seem to work. One bottle of cough syrup can cost upwards of $6 and might last a week if you are lucky or only have 1 sick person in the house, but what are the chances of that? By making your own remedies from the comfort of your own kitchen you can take the chill out of being sick and the sting out of your budget.

Allspice: Allspice can be brewed in a tea by steeping 1-2 teaspoons of the powdered berries per cup of boiling water for 10-20 minutes. Take up to 3 cups per day.

Angelica Cough syrup
1 handful Angelica root
1 quart of water
Boil down for 3 hours (gently)
Strain and add to honey
Take 2 tablespoons morning and night. (As well as throughout the day)
Anise: Just smell anise and you will be reminded of some of the over-the-counter cough remedies. Teas made from crushed seeds can soothe cold symptoms or anise can also be used to flavor syrups and lozenges.

Basil: Use in a tea, steam or cough medicines. You can also add basil to soup. I recommend chicken soup with basil, cayenne, rosemary and thyme. You can also use the juice of fresh basil leaves with honey or mix with elecampane and hyssop for coughs. The steam is great for head colds and the juice used in a decoction with cinnamon and clove will reduce chills.

Bayberry: You can use bayberry in teas with yarrow, catnip, sage or peppermint.

Benzoin: Inhale tincture steam. It doesn't smell very good but it will help with the congestion. You can use a vaporizer for this or if you don't have a vaporizer, place a pan of water on to boil and place a few drops of the tincture in the water. Do not let it boil dry.

Catnip: Catnip can soothe spasms caused by coughing fits and ease tension. Use as a tea or a tincture with Boneset, *Elder, *Yarrow or Cayenne.

Cayenne: You know when you eat spicy food how your eyes can start to water and you nose starts to run? That's the idea behind using cayenne. Added to foods or soups cayenne helps to clear nasal passages as well as speed up circulation and promote sweating which can help to break a fever.

Cinnamon: Drink an infusion to relieve cold and flu symptoms.

Echinacea: May be taken in capsules or drank in a tea. It should be used daily for the prevention of cold/flu. If taken at the onset of cold/flu symptoms Echinacea will cut the life of the cold short. Use with Goldenseal as a tincture.

Elder: Use the flowers or berries alone or with Peppermint,*Yarrow or Hyssop in a tea or tincture for colds and fevers, for flu use with Boneset.

Eucalyptus: Use the oil in lozenges or cough drops or for

steam inhalant for congestion. Mix 2 drops Eucalyptus oil with 2 drops Peppermint oil and 2 drops Tea Tree oil   or   1 fresh sprig of *Rosemary (keep eyes closed and breath deeply for 3 minutes). Also used as a vapor bath. The tincture works well for chest colds.

Evening primrose oil: This lovely night blooming flower holds a well-deserved place in the kitchen. As useful as it is beautiful the primrose can be used as a decoction of the root to make cough syrups or teas.

Garlic: Is a potent antibiotic that when taken or eaten can keep colds away. It can also be used as an expectorant and for sinus problems.

Ginger: The spicy root of ginger can be used for a number of things including to relieve and combat cold symptoms. Use it alone or with other herbs.

Juniper: When smoldered on a charcoal burner juniper clears congestion. Juniper may be substituted by Cedar.

Lavender: Use a few drops of the oil in a warm bath with 2 tablespoons of milk or cream to ease the body aches.

Lemon: Helps to fight colds and flu. It is packed with vitamin C and can make some teas go down a little easier. Add 1 squeezed lemon wedge with 1 teaspoon of honey to teas or drink lemonade to help stay hydrated during your illness.

Linden: Another ingredient that can be used with *Elder flower

Marshmallow: Boil the powdered root in milk or wine to make into syrup for coughs. This is the easiest way for children to swallow the medicine. The powdered root is also a key ingredient for making lozenges.

Mullein: Use a steam inhalant of Mullein for congestion and the tea is use for clearing the lungs.

Olive: Use the leaf extract to kill the cold virus and bacteria.

Pennyroyal: The leaves of this sweet mint plant can be made in to a tea to help with cold and flu symptoms as well as headache.

Peppermint: Drink peppermint tea to sooth coughs and congestion. Breathe deep while you sip it. You can also use peppermint oil in lozenges. At bedtime try putting a few drops on your pillow to help relax your airways.

Red Clover: Can be used in a tea or cough syrup to reduce coughing.

Rosemary: You can add a sprig of rosemary to boiling water and inhale the steam for congestion. Also use rosemary tea as an expectorant for cold and flu symptoms. Be sure to preserve the steam while making. Rosemary can be used in broth as well.

Sage: Particularly white sage can be infused for colds. This is especially useful when the cold is accompanied by a headache.

Sweet Marjoram: Use 1-2 teaspoons of the herb and flowers to make a tea or broth. Steep for 10 minutes and drink 3 times a day.

Thyme: Thyme has many flavored varieties such as caraway thyme and lemon thyme. We usually use common thyme to cook with but some of the flavored hybrids   may be more preferable for medicinal use. Use the thyme of your choice as a tea or broth for coughs or add to soups. Lemon thyme is usually best for treating children.

Chest cold tea

1 part anise seed
2 parts coltsfoot leaves
2 parts Lungwort
Steep 2 teaspoons on mix in ½ cup boiling water,
Add resulting tea to 1 ½ cups of Althea tea (see below),
Take mixture with honey in mouthful doses.

Althea tea

Soak 1 tablespoon Althea root, leaves and/or flowers in ½ cup
cold water for 8 hours.

St. John's wort tea for coughs

1 part St. Johns wort
½ part thyme
½ part linden flower
1 teaspoon mixture per cup water steep 5-10 minutes. Sweeten
with honey.

Yerba Mate: The tea can help boost the immune system as well
as work as an antioxidant against the cold and flu virus.

Fever

A fever is a way that the body fights off infection, but if
left untreated or if it goes to high it can cause real damage. For
low-grade fevers that are accompanied by body aches and stiff
muscles use these remedies in combination with those listed
under pain. For moderate to high fevers cool the skin with
lukewarm water and use these remedies to keep the fever down.
For extremely high fevers (over 104 degrees) or fevers that will
not respond to treatment seek medical attention immediately.

Angelica: Use in an infusion to lower a fever.

1 quart water
6 ounces Angelica root sliced thin
4 ounces honey
The juice of 2 lemons
½ gill of brandy
Infuse for ½ hour and drink.

Basil: Use tea made with basil and peppercorns to reduce fever. This mixture can also be placed in chicken broth.

Bayberry: Use as a fever reducer tea or decoction 1 teaspoon powdered root in 1 pint of hot water. Steep 10-15 minutes then add a bit of milk and cool to drink.

Belladonna: The root is used in some fever reducing remedies, (but an overdose can be fatal.) In tinctures use no more than 5-15 drops (made from root or leaves) in powdered form 1-2 grains for leaves or 1-5 grains for roots.

Catnip: Use fresh or dried herbs for tea. Helps bring down fever fast plus it is safe and pleasant tasting.

Cinnamon: Use the oil or cinnamon sticks to create a soothing tea.

Echinacea: Can be made into a tea or taken as capsules.

Feverfew: Just as the name suggests it lessens a fever. Feverfew can be chewed or drank as a tea. Chewing feverfew may cause irritation. If it does you should use as a tea or take as capsules.

Ginger: Promotes sweating when eaten which can help to eliminate fevers.

Willow: When chewed or brewed in a tea white willow bark reacts just like aspirin.

Yarrow: Can be used with Elder flower, Peppermint, Boneset, Cayenne and Ginger

Fever Reducer Tea

1 tsp dried Yarrow
1 tsp dried Elderflower
2 cups hot water
Drink ¼ cup per every ½ hour as needed.

Fever Tea #2

2 teaspoons dried sage
1 teaspoon dried peppermint
1 cup hot water
Steep covered for 15 minutes strain and sweeten with honey
Sip warm up to 3 cups per day

Fever Tea #3

1½ cups water
1 teaspoon dried fenugreek seeds
1 teaspoon thyme
¼ teaspoon powdered cayenne
Bring water to a boil, add fenugreek, reduce heat and simmer
for 5 minutes
Place thyme in a teapot, pour the unstrained fenugreek
decoction over it, cover and steep for 10 minutes. Strain and
stir in cayenne. Sweeten with honey sip warm.

Sore throat

Allergies, sinus trouble or just talking too much can cause a raw, scratchy, irritated throat. If your throat dries out at night while you're sleeping, it may be keeping your partner awake too.

Aloe Vera: You can use the juice as a gargle to soothe irritated throats and combat any bacteria or infection that might be building up.

Bayberry: If you have strep throat or tonsillitis use a gargle with a bayberry decoction to reduce inflammation.

Basil: Drink basil as a tea or a broth. You can also gargle with it. Mix 10 drops basil tincture with 2 tablespoons lemon juice and ¼ teaspoon salt in 1 cup of warm water.

Caraway: The seeds can be used for the treatment of laryngitis. Use as a gargle.

Echinacea: You can use an Echinacea tincture as a mouthwash to help fight off germs and bacteria.

Fennel: An infusion of the seeds can be used as a gargle to treat sore or irritated throats.

Ginger: A tea of ginger can be used as a gargle.

Hawthorn: Use the decoction 10-15 drops taken a few times a day.

Lemon: A lemon wedge can be used to make a gargle for sore throat. Squeeze or bite into the lemon and gargle with the fresh juice.

Raspberry: Use the leaves to make a strong tea to use as a gargle.

Sage: Can be used as a gargle for sore throats and tonsils.

Thyme: Use your favorite flavor of thyme to make a tea and use as a gargle. Lemon thyme works best for kids.

<u>Whooping cough</u>

One of the worst sounding coughs you will ever hear, the whooping cough is signified by a barking like croup. Those affected by whooping cough often experience other discomforts such as: raw irritated throats, chest and stomach spasms, headache, and shortness of breath. Treating the cough is the main focus but do not forget to treat the rest of the body as well. Symptoms like anxiety, depression and stress may not show up on the surface but can complicate the healing process.

Anise: Make a tea from the crushed anise seeds or use them to add flavor to a cough syrup.

Bayberry: Use the tea as a gargle then swallow it to break up the phlegm.

Garlic: The cloves of garlic crushed with cayenne pepper and honey can be used to clear the throat. Inhale the vapors of the freshly expressed juice, dilute with equal parts   water.

Lobelia: A few drops of the oil can be taken internally every few minutes as needed.

Red Clover: Drink as an infusion or use to flavor cough syrups.

Thyme: Combines with well with Wild cherry and Sundew.

Wild Cherry Bark: Can be used to make a tea or cough syrup.

Whooping cough tea #1

1 part Sundew
1 part Fennel
3 parts Primrose flower
5 parts Thyme
Steep 1 teaspoon of mixture in ½ cup boiling water for 3-5 minutes,
Add 1 teaspoon honey
Take 1-1 ½ cups a day in mouthful doses

Whooping cough tea #2

European mistletoe
Sage
Soak 2 teaspoons mistletoe in ½ cup cold water for 6-8 hours,
Steep 2 teaspoons sage in 1 cup boiling water, strain and let cool
Add mistletoe tea and take mouthful dose unsweetened as needed.

Eyes

If the eyes truly are the windows to the soul, or even if they are not, they are often the first thing people see when they look at us so we want to make sure they are clear. The eyes can tell a lot about how we are feeling both physically and mentally. Before using any eyewash, remove your contact lenses.

Aloe Vera: Use the juice as an eyewash. This may help to protect the eyes from UV   damage.

Bilberry: Also known as European blueberry can be eaten to promote healthy eyes and   reduce bloodshot eyes. This can also be replaced with blueberries or cranberries for the same benefits.

Calendula: Also known as pot marigold can be used to soothe irritated eyes. Use the tea to make a compress for eyes.

Chamomile: Use 1 drop of the oil on cool damp cotton ball applied to the eyes for 10 minutes. Keep your eyes closed. This works on tired and puffy eyes. This is also good for pink eye, otherwise known as conjunctivitis.

Fennel: Use 1 drop of fennel oil on a cool damp cotton ball for sore eyes. Keep eyes closed.

Watermelon seed: When eating a watermelon don't just spit the seeds out, chew them up and swallow them. No, a watermelon will not grow in your belly but your eyes will certainly benefit from this. Watermelon seeds work to promote healthy eyes and they are a natural antioxidant.

Wild Cherry Bark: Use a cold infusion as an eyewash.

<u>Eye Shake</u>

1 cup soy/skim milk
1 dash cinnamon
1 tbsp flax seed oil
1 tbsp lecithin granules
2 scoops whey protein
½ banana or 1 cup fresh (frozen) fruit
Add ice, blend all together and drink.

Hair loss

Though they say; "Bald is beautiful" some people are not yet ready to embrace a bare head. Millions of men and women are face with thinning hair and thousand of dollars a year are spent trying to stop or reverse the process. These are some natural and inexpensive ideas for the treatment and prevention of balding or thinning hair. These are not guaranteed to re-grow hair but anything is possible.

Aloe Vera: You can crush pieces of the fresh plant or buy commercially prepared products with aloe in them. Gently massage the gel on to head and scalp. It helps to stimulate the hair follicles and it feels good too. Rinse after about 5 minute.

Rosemary: Massage Rosemary oil into scalp or soak 1 cup fresh herb in 2 cups warm water bring to a gentle boil, then let stand covered for 1 hour. Strain herbs and mix water with 2 cups fresh cold water and use as a final rinse after shampooing. You can also mix an infusion of rosemary with Borax and use cold or place sprigs of rosemary with sprigs of mint in vinegar in a bottle with a tight lid. Put in a dark place for about 1 week before use.

Yarrow: Pick the fresh flowers to wash head with. You can also use the oil or an infusion of yarrow. This is only for the prevention of baldness it will not help to re-grow hair.

Hair loss
1 part nettle leaves
1 part onion
100 parts 70% alcohol
Soak the leaves and the onion in the alcohol for several days then massage into the scalp daily.

Regular stimulation of the hair follicles can not only encourage hair growth, but it works well for relieving tension. Store brand hair oils with ginseng can work to nourish the scalp as well as condition the hair, you may want to apply it with a head massager or just use your bare hands. Better yet use someone else's hands. A good head massage can stimulate intimacy as well.

Hiccoughs

Hiccoughs are not dangerous but they are very annoying and anything that gets rid of them fast is a relief, other than holding your breath or drinking tons of water, both of which can be uncomfortable.

Dill: Just take 2-3 big sniffs. It works that quickly but you can repeat as needed. You can   also eat a dill pickle.

Honey: (or sugar) eat one teaspoon. Repeat if needed. For infants place the honey or   sugar in a warm bottle of water. Do not use honey with newborns.

Lemon: Suck on a lemon wedge for a few seconds.

Peanuts: Eating a spoonful of peanut butter can eliminate the hiccoughs.

Immune system

The immune system is the first line of defense, other than the skin, in the battle against illness. If the immune system is weak or over-taxed, we are susceptible to just about any germ or bug that may invade. It is easier to avoid sickness or to shorten the length of any illness if we keep our immune system strong and healthy.

American Ginseng: A milder form of the popular Asian formula, American Ginseng can be used in teas or in capsules to help strengthen the immune system.

Cat's claw: New research shows an increased demand for cat's claw to aid in many immune functions. It can be taken to boost the immune system as well as a variety of other benefits.

Echinacea: When used with Goldenseal and vitamin C, Echinacea is a very strong immune system booster. It can be found in most heath teas and herbal supplements. It is a lovely addition to any garden as well.

Evening primrose oil: EPO has shown a number of health benefits when it is taken internally. Though it is probably well worth the money EPO can be quite costly.

Green tea: Has many healing benefits both internally and externally. Green tea can be taken daily as a capsule or as a refreshing drink. If you happen to get hurt while drinking green tea, just pour a little bit on the wound to clean it, or on a clean cloth and place it on the wound to stop any infection from setting in.

Licorice: The root not the candy can be chewed or used in teas, tinctures and astringents.

St. John's Wort: Other than its benefits to emotional balance, St. John's wort can be used to fight off infections. It makes a great ointment or lotion for preventing skin irritations from turning infected.

Yerba Mate: Helps to boost the energy as well as the immune system without the use of Ephedra.

Infection

Infections can be internal causes of illness or external wounds. Either way any infection must be handled quickly to prevent further complications. Internal infections may show up accompanied by fever or excessive amounts of discolored mucus. External infections around a wound are most likely seen with redness or fever around the area with a possible discharge or oozing.

Apple cider vinegar: When taken internally can fight off infection from the inside. It can also be used externally to treat wounds and skin abrasions.

Echinacea: Can be taken internally and fights most kinds of infections.

Garlic: When eaten daily fights most forms of microbial infection, combines well with Echinacea. Garlic can also be applied to wounds to kill off any external infections due to bacteria.

Kelp: A member of the seaweed family, kelp is a healthy natural defense as well as a good source of calcium and fiber.

Lavender: The essential oil of lavender can prevent infection in minor skin irritations. Just place a few drops right on the wound. This also helps with the stinging so kids don't mind it as much.

Myrrh: Can be used externally with Witch Hazel as an ointment, cream, or astringent to fight off bacterial infections.

Rose Hips: Roses are grown just about everywhere. You don't have to spend a lot of money at a florist to get them. Some grow wild and can be easily transplanted to your own garden. Legend has it they grow best when taken wild from the land of another (this is not to say that I condone theft). The rose hip is just one of the many useful parts of this lovely fragrant plant. Water made from rose hips can be used to clean wound areas.

Worms

When is a worm not a worm? When it's a virus. Ringworm is only listed in this section because it is commonly thought of as a worm and some of the same remedies that treat actual worm infestations such as tapeworm or round worms can also work for the treatment of ringworm.

Basil: Drink tea to expel intestinal worms, but use the leaf juice with honey externally for ringworm.

Black walnut: Use the nut including the green hull externally to kill ringworm and tapeworms.

Garlic: The clove is crushed and applied to the area externally, eaten it kills the internal worms.

Lemongrass: The fresh crushed herb can be applied to ringworm.

Mugwort: The infusion can encourage the expulsion of worms. It is also an antiseptic that can be used to treat malaria.

Tea Tree Oil: Can be used directly on the area.

Kidneys

The kidneys work to filter out impurities and toxins in the blood stream. We don't always take care of our kidneys the way we should, overloading our systems with caffeine and not taking in enough water and nutrients to help maintain proper function. When we neglect our kidneys they can become infected and or damaged. Early indications of this can range from mild to sever lower back pain to fever and jaundice.

Diuretics

The excess fluids that are kept in the body can cause swelling, discomfort, and even pain. Most of the extra weight that we want to lose (like that last 10 pounds) comes from water weight. Though it is important to stay hydrated, too much water can actually flush out important electrolytes. New research now shows that 4-5 glasses of water a day under normal circumstances are sufficient to maintain healthy hydration. More water is required during times of high heat and physical activity. The water intake should be balance with the replenishment of electrolytes, sodium and potassium that may be lost during physically demanding sports or other activities.

Angelica: There are many ways to enjoy Angelica. A tea made of Angelica can stimulate kidney function, but the other parts of the plant are tasty too.

Basil: Cooking with basil is funny; you never have enough until you have too much. It's a good thing it is so useful. Basil can be added to just about any food or used in teas and broths.

Benzoin: Can be taken internally as an infusion or tincture. It tastes and smells funny but is worth it.

Celery seed: Can be eaten with your favorite foods or made into a tea. Try using celery salt in place of regular table salt to give some of your favorite recipes a neat new flavor.

Dandelion: And you thought it was just an annoying little weed. Dandelions can be used with Couchgrass or Yarrow for water retention. You can also make a tea from the dandelion leaves, roots or flowers.

Dandelion Teas
4 or 5 flowers added to warm water and brought to a slow boil for 3-4 minutes.
The dried or fresh leaves and/or roots steeped in hot water covered for 5 minutes.

Dandelion salad
Fresh young dandelion leaves mixed with salad greens, celery seeds, and balsamic or (apple cider vinegar) dressing

Elder: The flowers can be drunk as a tea to clear toxins from the body.

Juniper: The berries made into a tea or added to foods work as a diuretic. Juniper can be crushed and used as a rub for poultry, or whole berries added to stews, soups or beans.

Kava: Can be taken as capsules or used in a tea.

Marshmallow: Use the root in a tea. Just don't boil it too long or it will become thick.

Mullein: The tea is a great diuretic as well as a liver tonic. Can be use as an infusion as well.

Diuretic tea

Asparagus root
Fennel root
Celery root
Parsley root

Mix in equal parts and steep 1 teaspoon in ½ cup boiling water. Take ½ to 1 cup per day unsweetened in mouthful doses.

Kidneys

Used in combination with good nutrition and diuretics, these remedies concentrate on maintaining proper kidney function to ensure better overall health.

Alfalfa: When alfalfa is eaten it keeps the kidneys healthy and functioning properly. Alfalfa sprouts can be added to salads, sandwiches, and wraps.

Basil: As well as being used for diuretic purposes, basil can be eaten or taken in teas and broths to maintain kidney health.

Celery seed: With an interestingly slightly bitter after taste, a little bit of these little seeds can go a long way. Celery seeds can be eaten or taken in a tea or celery salt used in many recipes.

Clove: Spicy and sweet the powerful clove can be added to most any food from meats to baked goods. The oil can also be used to flavor foods and beverages.

Dong quai: Besides the beauty it will bring to your garden, Dong quai strengthens the kidneys when taken internally. It is incredibly versatile. Experiment with different ways to eat the shoots, buds and leaves.

Sage: White sage can be used to stimulate the kidneys and to eliminate toxins.

Urinary tract

The burning of a urinary tract infection can be very disturbing. There are a few things you may have in the house that can ease the pain and inflammation at least until you can see a doctor.

Bayberry: Can be taken internally for the treatment of the infection, use with Echinacea and the common lawn weed Plantain.

Cranberry: Sweet simple cranberry juice. Drink a glass or two every day to stop the infection or use some of the berries as part of your normal diet. You can also use   the pills if you are worried about your sugar intake. By taking cranberry you could be able to stop infections caused by E. coli

Marshmallow: Use the leaves made into a tea to help stop the infection or make a marshmallow syrup to take daily for kidney and urinary tract health.

Kids

When children get sick the whole family can feel the pain and discomfort. From late night coughing spasms to vomiting and diarrhea a sick child can be irritable and most parents find it very difficult to comfort them. Though most remedies are safe for children in diluted or smaller doses, these are specifically geared for the kids. They are made with not only the symptom but also taste in mind. After all a remedy will not work if you can't get them to take it. Some of these will work on even the most finicky of children. As well I have included some treats that even mom and dad will feel good about.

Anise: The seeds have a yummy candy smell and taste that most kids find easy to swallow. Use as a tincture or as a tonic for flatulent colic in infants.

Caraway: To use the seed oil as a tonic for flatulent colic. Apply 1-4 drops of oil on a sugar cube or in 1 teaspoon of water.

Caraway Julep

1 ounce bruised caraway seeds
1 pint of cold water
Infuse for 6 hours
1-3 teaspoons per dose for infants.

Catnip: Tasty enough for kiddies (and kitties like it too). The tincture or tea can be taken for diarrhea. Catnip also helps soothe irritability. Try the catnip snack recipe located in the digestion section for a healthy refreshing treat.

Cloves: Use an infusion for colic.

Evening primrose oil: EPO is used externally to control

hyperactivity. Rub EPO mixed with carrier oil on skin for infants and children. The roots or tops of the Evening primrose are naturally sweet and can be boiled in honey to make cough syrup.

Flax seed oil: This is excellent for use in all areas of growth, (bone, skin, muscle, brain, etc.) It is great for healthy teeth. Pour a little over oatmeal or try it as a salad dressing. Try the flax seed butter recipe located in the Heart Healthy section.

Fennel: Use the infusion as a safe treatment for children with colic or teething pain.

Red Clove: The same little flowers that we suckled honey out of as children can be made into a cough syrup or given as a tea for the treatment of croupy cough.

Safflower: Can be added to food or given as a tea. It aids in fighting Measles and fever. The steam is used for skin complaints like chicken pox or measles rashes.

Saffron: As a tea or in food saffron has a calming affect on infants and children especially during teething. It has also been used to sooth chicken pox. Use powdered saffron to make a paste and apply to the itchy area. This can be made fun if you let the children finger paint each other in the yellow paste.

High Calcium Tea for Kids

1 part each: 2 part each 3 parts 6 parts ½ parts
Nettle lemon balm rose hips fennel cinnamon
Oat straw mint
Raspberry leaf

Calming Tea for Kids

1 part oat straw 1 part rose petals
½ parts catnip 2 parts chamomile
1 part licorice root 2 parts linden flower
1 part slippery elm bark 2 parts mint

Respiratory Tonic Tea

1 part Red clover
1 part mullein
1 part coltsfoot
2 parts lemon balm
4 parts rose hips
4 parts fennel
1 part Calendula

Colic tea for infants

4 parts fennel seed
3 parts mint
2 parts chamomile flower
1 part valerian
Steep ½ teaspoon of the mixture in 1½ cups boiling water for 5
minutes.
Strain and give 5-6 doses during the day with warm milk or
alone.

Angelica candy

2 cups Angelica stems (young shoots)
2 cups boiling water
½ cup salt
Syrup is made with
2 cups sugar
2 cups water
1 tablespoon lemon juice

Place Angelica in a large bowl and cover with salt and water. Let set covered with a towel for 1 day. Drain, peel and rinse in cool water. Cook sugar and water to syrup stage (about 240 degrees F). Add Angelica and lemon juice and cook another 20 minutes stirring often. Drain off the stems (reserving the syrup in the refrigerator) and place Angelica on a rack in a cool dark place for 3-4 days. Return syrup and Angelica to the pot and cook about 15-20 minutes or until candied. Drain Angelica and store on a rack until dry then store in a sealed jar.

Diaper rash

Babies have very sensitive skin and when it is irritated by diaper rash it can make for a very unhappy camper. To help keep baby happy and healthy (as well as mom) it is best to treat the problem at the first signs of redness or irritation. It is a good idea to change the diaper often and to keep the diaper area clean and dry.

Aloe Vera: To soothe baby's bottom when irritation and redness occur use Aloe Vera gel. It can be applied to directly to the affected area.

Cinnamon: Use finely ground cinnamon mixed with equal or ¾ part cornstarch as a diaper powder. Cinnamon can be irritating to the skin, use to prevent but not on already irritated or sensitive skin. (Do not use cornstarch on yeast induced diaper rash)

Tea Tree Oil: Since tea tree oil is a strong anti everything, diaper rash is no problem. Mix about 25 drops of tea tree oil with gentle carrier oil and apply to affected areas.

Herbal salve

1 part St. John's Wort
1 part comfrey leaf and root

1 part Calendula
Use herbs or a tincture to make an ointment or cream to treat diaper rash.

Men's health

It's tough being the king of your castle. Men face a great deal of health issues today, though getting them to talk about them is not always easy. Among the major concerns men face are heart health, cancer, prostate health and libido. Though most of these topics have been covered in general in other sections, this section focuses on treatments specifically with the men in mind. One of the most important things a guy can do to stay healthy is unwind once in a while. Men carry a lot of internal burdens that they are not always comfortable talking about but if they will take a little time each day or even one day a week and treat themselves to something relaxing it can improve their health body and soul.

Libido

Bananas: Eating bananas will help to increase male libido and it's a good quick snack.

Basil: Adding basil to foods helps to promote healthy sexual function.

Clove: Add this sweet spice to your meals to increase blood flow and promote lust.

Garlic: Using garlic as well as its relatives, ginger, onion, leek and scallion, can have many wonderful benefits for sexual health.

Gingko: The nut can increase blood flow when eaten

Oat: Eating oats helps to release testosterone into the blood stream.

Spikenard: The oil extract of spikenard a relative on valerian root can be soothing. Use if stress is the cause of your dysfunction. 15 drop of oil mixed with a carrier base or mixed into a cream and used as a soothing massage.

Prostate health

Garlic: Eating garlic can enhance immune function and possible fight off cancer formation.

Green tea: Drinking green tea works to clean the system, as well it has shown to be beneficial when fighting cancer.

Soy: Soy products such as soy milk can keep the testosterone levels in balance as well as reduce the risk of cancer.

Tomatoes: Foods that are rich in Lycopene such as tomatoes, pink grapefruits and watermelon help to protect the cells from cancer. Cook the tomatoes for a higher concentration of Lycopene.

Testicular health

Basil: Adding basil to foods is an easy way to get a daily dose of this cancer fighting spice.

Chives: Helps to destroy tumor cells

Thyme: Works like basil in fighting cancer and can be added to most any foods.

Turmeric: One of the only herbs known to help expel carcinogens.

Mind

Health and healing involve mind and body. The fact is our state of mind may have a lot more to do with how often we get sick as well as how sever that illness is and how long it takes to recover. A healthy mind is the best place to start when dealing with any illness. Therefore, these remedies can and should be used in conjunction with remedies from every other section. As well you may keep a few of them on hand to use as preventative medicine.

Anxiety

At some point we all experience symptoms of anxiety. This kind of tension can be harmful to the body as well as the mind. The following remedies can help sooth jitters, nervousness, and hyperactivity associated with anxiety to help maintain a peaceful balance between mind and body.

Black Cohosh: Can be used in teas to soothe nerves and calm general restlessness. It is particularly useful with symptoms of menopause.

Bay: The leaves can be made into a tea to calm hysteria.

Catnip: Catnip has a very soothing affect on humans as well as on cats. Drinking tea made with catnip can calm nerves in adults and children and it is a good way to spend time with your cat too. That is if you don't mind sharing. You can also take a bath with the infusion of catnip as a great stress reducer at the end of a hard day.

Chamomile: These little daisy-like flowers are just as nice to look at as they are to use. I have found even the simple act of stirring a cup of chamomile tea can be soothing. It has a sweet aroma that is naturally calming. Drink 1 to 2 cups of the tea steeped for 10 minutes. It may be mixed with other herbs for increased benefit. The chamomile flowers can be added to salads and the petals are an edible decoration for cakes and cookies. Chamomile welcomes you home when planted near a walkway; its aroma is released with each step.

Evening primrose oil: This beautiful bright yellow flower is used in many different ways. The oil of the Evening primrose (EPO) comes from the seeds that can be boiled or roasted and used on salads or in bread. EPO improves the over all feeling of well-being. You can also eat the leaves as cooked greens, the flowers as a sweet treat on salads, and the root can be boiled like a potato only sweeter.

Ginger: Use the root to make teas, tinctures or in capsules to reduce anxiety.

Hops: The tincture can be used to reduce anxiety or the flowers can be placed in a pillow to help you sleep if you are restless at night.

Kava: The easiest way to get Kava is through a retailer such as a health and nutrition store that sells vitamins and herbal supplements. You should follow the directions on the bottle if you intend to take it this way.

Lavender: The oil mixed with carrier oil can be calming. The fresh flowers can add a soothing touch to the house.

Linden: This little yellow flower is a native of European trees. It's naturally sweet fragrance and flavor can be soothing for any disposition. Linden can be used with Hops in infusions, decoctions, teas and tinctures. Take 1 cup of tea every 2 hours.

Rosemary: Use the tincture to reduce stress.

Saffron: Though it is very expensive Saffron is very aromatic and is useful in many ways. Just its scent alone can be soothing. It has been a culinary delight for ages that can produce feelings of well being when eaten or added to milk. Try using some in your favorite baked goods.

Sage: White sage infusions can calm the nerves.

Skullcap: This little herb is a wonderful addition to any garden as well as an excellent remedy for nervousness. It helps to stop irritability associated with PMS or hormonal imbalances.

St. John's Wort: One of the best mood balancing herbs on the market. St. John's Wort can be used in teas or taken as capsules. St. John's Wort will combine well with mother's wort, lemon balm, and lavender

Sweet Marjoram: Not to be confused with common Oregano, the taste of Sweet marjoram is one of sweet and spicy. It can be used as a tea steeping the herb for 10 minutes in boiling water or in a broth if the taste does not suit you. It is also a nice addition to most recipes including meats, fish, poultries, eggs and soups. You can drink the tea or broth 3 times a day to sooth nerves. It is gentle enough for use on children.

Valerian: This stinky and bitter herb is one of best sedatives you can find. It can be used in teas, but you may want to mix it with something or just put it in capsule form. If you can handle the smell it is worth it for a good night of natural sleep. Cats love it too.

Calming Tea

1 part chamomile
½ part valerian
1 stick cinnamon
Add honey to taste

Soothing oils

3 drops lavender oil
1 drop anise oil
2 drops peppermint oil
Place in an infuser in your bedroom at bedtime,
or mix with baby oil and use as a massage oil.

Depression

Some days you just can't help but feel down. There are a lot of things that can contribute to the blues and the overwhelming feeling of depression such as stress, PMS, sickness and the weather. Sometimes depression can be a symptom of a more serious problem. Though we cannot always cure the cause of depression we can ease the symptoms and take heart in the fact that all things pass in time.

Basil: You can drink basil in a tea or used in a bath to relieve depression especially postpartum depression. It is also good when added to food. I would recommend a   nice warm bowl of soup or broth on a rainy day.

Celery seed: Can be used in tea and foods to aid with depression associated with arthritis.

Lavender: Combines with*Rosemary, Kola or Skullcap to form a soothing tea or inhalant. Lavender oil can be use in a diffuser, a bath or applied directly to the skin. Added to jasmine a few dabs on the wrist can be uplifting.

Oat: When mixed with Skullcap and Mugwort oat can restore balance. Try baking it into a batch of your favorite cookies.

Rosemary: Has a powerful affect on depression. It can be used in teas, broths, or in a bath. For baths, place a sprig of the fresh herb under the running faucet.

Saffron: Just the scent of this big purple flower with its prized yellow center can be enough to brighten your day. Saffron can be used in teas and in baked foods. The flavor is very uplifting. An infusion of saffron can also be used to make perfumes.

St. John's Wort: One of the most popular methods of treating depression, St. John's wort has shown to be effective on anxiety as well as depression. It works to balance out the moods not just elevate or lower them. Used in teas or taken as capsules can help regulate moods. It is most effective when taken over a period of time.

Squaw vine: This can be used as a treatment for depressions relating to female disorders such as postpartum depression or depression related to PMS.

Saffron Lavender Oatmeal cookies

2 eggs
½ cup margarine
1 cup sugar
1½ cups self-rising flour
1 cup quick oats
1 tsp lavender leaves
1 tsp saffron
Icing: confectioner's sugar and Rose water.
Preheat oven to 375 degrees. Use a blender to mix eggs, margarine, sugar, lavender and saffron. Place in a large mixing bowl and gradually add flour. Mix well and drop by the teaspoonful onto a non-greased cookie sheet. Bake until light brown. Mix together confectioner's sugar and rose water to form a smooth icing. Cover cookies with icing and let cool.

Lavender mint tea

2 parts dried mint
1 part dried lavender flower

Steep 1 teaspoon of mint per 1 cup of boiling water for 10 minutes.
Add ½ teaspoon lavender and let cool.

Yerba Mate: Use the tea to help reduce depression.

Memory

Whether it is an occasional bout of forgetfulness, or the early on set of diseases such as Alzheimer's or senility, our memories are precious. One might say they are the records of our lives. By taking means to stimulate our brains we can protect it and to some degree enhance its capability.

Ginkgo: Taking ginkgo biloba can increase memory loss and stimulate brain function. It has been show to also reduce the ringing in your ears. Ginkgo can be taken in a tea or capsules.

Kava: To increase mental alertness, memory and concentration Kava may be taken in tea or capsules.

Ginseng: American or otherwise, ginseng helps to balance brain functions and improve memory.

Flax seed: Taking flax seed oil can improve concentration and memory and has a significant affect on ADD/ADHD. The seeds or the oil can be added to recipes.

Rosemary: Eating food with rosemary or using it in teas can aid your memory and learning. Also eating foods that are high in carotenes can increase your mental ability. Such foods are generally brightly colored such as carrot, spinach, and blueberries but also include other foods such as fish.

Sleep

Getting a good nights sleep is probably one of the most important things we need to do in order to stay healthy. Our bodies need this time off to heal and repair itself after the stress and strain of a busy day. But sometimes sleep doesn't come easily. It is then that we should reach out to nature the most. The amount of sleep we get isn't as important as the quality of the sleep we get. If our sleep cycle is inhibited by drugs, chemicals, or stress, it can be as bad for us as not sleeping at all.

Hops: The same stuff used to make beer, these flowers combine with Valerian and Passion flower to produce a strong sleep tonic. Hops flowers are very powerful and should not be used with severe depression.

Kava: Can be use in a tea or capsules to promote sleep.

Lavender: The sweet essential oil can be placed in a diffuser in your bedroom or used in a bath before bedtime. Place a few drops on your pillow too.

Linden: Calms the mind and helps promote sleep. Linden also relieves insomnia and helps to relieve tension. Try making a tea from these flowers.

Valerian: Works very well when used with chamomile. Valerian promotes a safe and natural sleep. It will not interfere with REM   sleep or dreams.

Insomnia tea #1

1 part Valerian
2 parts St. John's Wort
3 parts Hops
5 parts Lavender flower

10 parts Primrose flower
Steep 1 ½ teaspoons mixture in ½ cup boiling water for 10 min.
When cool enough to drink add 1 teaspoon of honey.
Sip before bedtime.

Insomnia tea #2

3 parts Hops
2 parts Valerian
Steep1 teaspoon mix in ½ cup boiling water
Take ½ to 1 cup a day unsweetened in mouthful doses
Do not take for more than 2-3 weeks

Stress

Stress is something that cannot be avoided. Our lives are made up of good stress and bad stress, the difference being how we handle it. When our stress levels get too high it can cause any number of problems from headaches to sleeplessness. Too much stress can be generated from work, family and everything in between. It is important to keep our stress levels within tolerable levels; this means both good and bad stress.

American Ginseng: This mild form of ginseng works just as well in a tea or in capsules as its Asian cousins. Any of the ginseng family will work to reduce stress on the body and the mind.

Chamomile tea: Simple is good.

Lavender: The fragrant oil can be used with a diffuser or in bath. Also the flowers can be added to beverages and foods for a relaxing treat.

Oats: Oatmeal is almost as simple as it gets. Oats can be eaten or placed in a bath. Mixed   with Mugwort, Oats are a heart healthy stress reducer.

Rose: Ever wonder why people almost always bring home roses after a fight? Roses can reduce stress and ease tension. Use the oil in a diffuser or dried rose hips, leaves and petals in a tea. A rose water bath can reduce stress as well.

St. John's Wort: Psychology in the garden, better known as herbal Prozac it works as well on stress and anxiety as it does on depression. Use in tea or capsules to help maintain balanced moods.

Valerian: Use valerian in any tea to help stay calm. Believe it or not cats like it too. (Caution Valerian is very stinky and bitter; you may consider mixing it with something like Chamomile and a little honey).

For insomnia due to stress

2 parts Dill seed
2 parts Anise seed
1 part Chamomile
1 part *Hops
Steep 1 teaspoon in ½ cup boiling water,
When lukewarm add 1 teaspoon of honey,
Sip before bedtime.

Stress tea

2 parts St. John's wort
1 part lemon balm
1 part valerian
1 tsp mix per cup boiling water for 10 minutes and drink before bed sweetened with honey.

Motherhood

Aside from the health issues women face there are special concerns for women who are or are thinking about becoming a mother. A lot of over the counter remedies can be harmful during pregnancy but that doesn't stop the need for those remedies. There are also concerns that are specific to fertility, pregnancy and childbirth that women must deal with, such as nutrition, lactation, pain and discomfort.

Childbirth
Childbirth should be a special time, but all too often it is an uncomfortable one as well. These are some ways to ensure a safe and healthy delivery that is reduced in pain and discomfort. Some of the remedies should not be taken during pregnancy itself but at time of delivery.

Angelica: The sweet angelica herb should be taken during labor and delivery. Use 1 tsp of the herb per cup boiling water to help if the delivery or post-delivery is difficult.

Basil: Can be used to stop postpartum hemorrhaging. It also makes a good tea or broth for the symptoms of postpartum depression. It can be used to help expel the placenta when used with a mother's wort infusion.

Black cherry: Drink Black cherry juice for relief from pain.

Blue Cohosh: It is one of the few herbs that can be taken at any point during the pregnancy to ensure an easy delivery as well as help with the threat of miscarriage.

Feverfew: Is used for difficult labor and after birth expulsion but should not be taken prior to labor.

Myrrh: Can be applied to navel after the cord is removed.

Raspberry: The leaves can be used in a tea to aid with uterine cramps as well as morning sickness. Use with ginger for extra relief.

Witch Hazel: Either the fresh plant leaves, branches and bark or the same stuff you buy in the store can be used as an astringent to treat bruising of the vulva and give relief of vaginal tenderness. It can be used as a compress or as a gentle cleanser.

Lactation
Milk production after a child is born is not always just a matter of waiting for the milk to come down. Sometimes there can be a shortage of this life giving food or an over abundance that lacks nutrients. During lactation it is important for mothers to eat healthy and be especially careful of what they take. Whatever she ingests will be passed to the baby through the breast milk.

Anise: Eating the sweet seeds will increase milk secretion. They can be added to foods or taken in teas and tonics.

Fennel: Fennel seeds taste and smell much like anise. Theses fragrant and flavorful seeds will increases the flow of milk.

Lemon grass: The essential oils from lemon grass can help to stimulate milk flow. Though the neat (or straight) oil can cause irritation to skin and should not be used on infants and children the fresh lemony scent can be soothing as well as up lifting. Use with carrier oils.

Squaw vine: Has been used by American Indians to increase milk flow as well as for breast health and enhancement.

Tea for nursing mothers
Anise seed

Dill seed
Sweet marjoram
Mix in equal parts and steep 1 teaspoon in ½ cup boiling water.
Take 1-1½ cups in mouthful doses per day, sweeten with honey.

Pregnancy
For some people getting pregnant is not as easy as it is for others. If we do get pregnant we want to do everything possible to ensure a healthy and problem free experience for ourselves as well as our children. Other than some of the more common problems that could arise during pregnancy, this section also includes some prenatal and fertility remedies.

Alfalfa: Increasing use of alfalfa sprouts can aid in reproduction for both men and women.

Blue Cohosh: One of the best things to take during any point of your pregnancy, blue cohosh aids in the prevention of miscarriage, eases false labor pain and dysmenorrhoea, and helps to ensure an easy delivery.

Catnip: This is a soothing tea that, among other things helps to prevent miscarriage and premature births.

Cayenne: Adding cayenne to your diet can help with the reproductive organs.

Cramp bark: As well as easing cramps, cramp bark can protect against miscarriage.

Ginseng: Taking ginseng can lower stress levels that can lead to infertility.

Raspberry: The leaves made into a tea will promote uterine health and alleviate pain. Drink raspberry tea in preparation for pregnancy as well as during to prevent complications.

Saw Palmetto: Regular use of saw palmetto can increase your chance of getting pregnant by strengthening the reproductive organs.

Squaw vine: Drinking teas made with squaw vine can help to prepare the body for child bearing.

Wild Yam: The root can be taken as capsules but the progesterone is hard for the body to break down and use so it is recommended to use in a cream form.

*Note:
Some herbs should be used from the beginning of menstruation until ovulation such as Black cohosh, and EPO or Flax seed oil. Others such as wild yam should be used from ovulation until menstruation. If you are trying to conceive, both men and women should stay away from St. John's wort, Echinacea and gingko biloba because they may inhibit fertility.

<u>Pregnancy tea</u>

Use for the prevention of nausea, miscarriage, and pain and to increase milk production.
1 part cinnamon
5 parts blackberry leaves
5 parts milfoil
10 parts raspberry leaves
Steep 1 teaspoon of mixture in ½ cup boiling water
Take ½ to 1 cup in mouthful doses daily.

Nose bleeds

There are many reasons why some people get nosebleeds. The most obvious of course is due to injury. But for the times when the nose starts bleeding and there are no signs of trauma it could simply be a matter of dryness. Keeping the nasal passageways clear and moist can be a key factor in preventing frequent nosebleeds.

Nettle: Once the herb has been dried and the stingers fall off, nettle can be made into an astringent and used to stop bleeding.

Witch Hazel: This is a common astringent found in most local stores. Witch hazel can be used to stop the bleeding and to clean the nasal passages safely and gently.

Yarrow: A tincture of yarrow can also be used as an astringent.

Salt water: A simple saline or salt-water solution will keep the membranes moist and prevent them for cracking and bleeding. You can make this one yourself by mixing ¼ teaspoon regular table salt with warm water. You will need to make a fresh mixture every day.

Pain

Pain is a fact of life. There are specific types of pain such as arthritis as well as general non-specific joint and muscle aches. Some prescription pain relievers can have adverse side effects while others may be habit forming. It seems every day there is yet another law suite involving a major drug company because a drug previously thought to be safe has now been discovered to be deadly. The thought of it can be scary or even overwhelming at times, but I believe that nature knows best. Even if a natural herbal remedies seems to take longer to be effective, in the long run I would much rather it be slow and safe than to be quick and deadly.

Arthritis:

The pain, swelling, and stiffness attributed to arthritis, rheumatism, and gout can be alleviated using a combination of internal and external remedies. Warm poultices and compresses can be used externally for specific painful areas while taking remedies internally can help reduce inflammation and fluid build up.

Alfalfa: A lot of people get a strange look on their face when I suggest that they eat alfalfa. It's not just for livestock you know. Alfalfa sprouts are a neat addition to   a n y salad or sandwich. When eaten alfalfa works from the inside out to promote healthy joints, or can also be used as a compress or poultice placed directly on the   affected area. Make a tea from the leaf.

Allspice: The sweet everything flavors of allspice contains a powerful pain reliever in its little dark berries. The crushed berries are boiled down to form a thick liquid that is then spread on the affected area as a poultice.

Aloe Vera: Dinking aloe juice works from the inside while the gel can be applied to the area to cool and soothe the joints.

Angelica: Yet another one of the multiple uses of this sweet and beautiful flower. The dried yellow juice of the Angelica plant can be taken as a medicine for pain and inflammation.

Apple cider vinegar: The added benefit of calcium and potassium in apple cider vinegar works wonders to ease the pain of arthritis and helps the body to heal itself. Just   mix   2 teaspoons of apple cider vinegar with 2 teaspoons of honey in a glass of water and drink 3 times a day. You can also use ¼ cup apple cider vinegar mixed with 1½ cups warm water as a soak or a poultice for stiff and painful areas.

Bayberry: Also known as Waxberry, this candle making plant offers a natural source of anti-inflammatory medication. The tea or decoction of leaves can be used for many ailments.

Belladonna: Also known as deadly nightshade can be used but only with extreme care and caution. The diluted tincture is used in a poultice or a lotion to lessen pain (use very small doses about ¼ —1 drop per dose). Or better yet use a remedy that is not as toxic.

Benzoin: The gum from the Benzoin tree can be made into a tincture massaged through the skin as a treatment for pain.

Cayenne: This spicy little pepper can be used as a poultice. Cayenne confuses the painful area and provides temporary relief. It is the primary ingredient in the well-known arthritis drug capsaicin.

Celery seed: The warm little seeds with the great big flavor and just a bit of bitter after taste though are an interesting addition to any meal, salad or dressing. When eaten the seeds work as a diuretic to reduce painful swelling and symptoms of arthritis as well as associated depression. Use as an infusion to treat arthritis pain. Use a tincture for rheumatism.

Chamomile: This sweet and tasty plant can make you feel good inside and out. The soothing oil and extracts are used for inflammation while the tea helps with the mental stress. Chamomile flowers can be place in a cloth with some powdered milk and added to a warm bath.

Devil's claw: Though it may be difficult to find and may not work in all cases it is said that Devil's claw is well worth it. It can be used with Bogbean, Celery seed or Meadowsweet to reduce inflammation.

Evening primrose oil: EPO works internally and is most

effective, but it is not without its drawbacks. For one it is very expensive and you need to take up to 12 pills at a time. There are other oils that are less costly and can be substituted for EPO, such as Flaxseed oil, nut oils, safflower oil and fish oils. Use 2 tablespoons of the alternate oils or ½ teaspoon of EPO per day.

Nettle: The stingers of the nettle may be used much like bee therapy in that you allow yourself to be stung by the plant directly on the affected area. I am not that big a fan of pain, especially when I already hurt, so I would recommend the use of nettle in a tea. The stingers will fall off during the drying process and the remaining leaves may be infused or uses as a tincture or decoction to be taken several times daily.

Arthritis poultice

6 parts Mullein leaves
9 parts Slippery elm bark
3 parts Lobelia
1 part Cayenne
Add 3 ounces of mixture to enough boiling water to form a paste. Spread on a cloth and apply to the swollen and painful joints.

Earache

An earache may be a warning sign that something else is wrong or it could be a side effect of some other ailment, such as a toothache or sinus infection. It is important to treat the whole problem. Use these remedies in combination with others to treat the whole problem.

Echinacea: Make an infusion or tincture of Echinacea combined with Ribwort (also known as plantain) and take orally.

Garlic: Use 2 drops of garlic oil placed on a cotton ball and put in the ear overnight.

Ginger: Instill 2-4 drops of warm ginger juice in the ear 2 times a day. This may also be done with radish juice.

Goldenseal: Take capsules or tincture internally or use 10ml of tincture to 100ml of water solution as eardrops.

Mullein: Use the cold infused oil as eardrops.

Warm (not hot) olive oil mixed with a few drops of lobelia oil and mullein oil and placed in the ear with a dropper. Place a small piece of cotton in the ear. Place a warm poultice made with a baked onion over the ear and rest.

Headache (migraines)

There are many reasons we get headaches and migraines though once they have set in we don't much care why. It is important to understand the cause of the headache to insure we are treating the right thing. For instance, you would not treat a sinus headache the same way you would treat a tension headache. Use these remedies in conjunction with others to treat the whole body.

Aloe Vera: The juice can be drunk to ease general headache pain.

Basil: Drink as a tea, or use powder as a snuff to stop a headache (though it may cause you to sneeze). Basil can also be added to food.

Bay: Another of those crazy herbs that you can never have enough of until you have too much. Bay leaves can be added to food or brewed in a tea. It can be combined with feverfew. It works on migraines too.

Feverfew: Can be chewed, used in capsules or as a tea. Drink it cold.

Hops: Makes a nice tea but can cause you to become sleepy. This works well for a headache at bedtime.

Lavender: The oil can be rubbed in at the temples especially for stress headaches.

Linden: Helps to relieve tension and reduce sinus headaches.

Pennyroyal: The sweet mint flavored leaves can be brewed into a tea for general headaches.

Peppermint: Mixed with carrier oil and rubbed on the temples will relieve a headache.

Rose: Soak a cloth in cold rose water and place on temples.

Rosemary: Used in a tea or as a steam inhalant for sinus headaches. Rosemary can be used in a bath to relieve tension headaches.

Saffron: Apply as a paste to the forehead. Saffron paste is quite good for your skin too.

Sweet Marjoram: Drink in a tea 3 times a day for the prevention of headaches.

Thyme: Use as a steam inhalant.

Willow: The bark can be chewed or brewed in tea. It will works like aspirin.

Headache tea

Chamomile
Valerian
Willow bark
Skullcap
Wood betony
Infuse in equal parts or use as a tincture.

Migraine tea

2 parts St. John's Wort
1 part Valerian
1 part Linden flower
¼ part crushed Juniper berry
Use 1 teaspoon of mix per cup of boiling water. Steep for 10 minutes, strain and sweeten.

Muscles

Over worked and stressed muscles can result from sports or work activities. A pulled or strained muscle can keep you off your feet and out of the game for several days. These remedies will help you to feel better and speed healing.

Alfalfa: Alfalfa is considered to be the athlete's wonder food. It promotes healthy bone, joint and muscle growth. Use as a poultice for sore or tired muscles.

Allspice: The crushed berries make a good compress or poultice for achy muscles. The oil of the allspice berry can be used as an anesthetic.

Celery seeds: These tiny little seeds are generally eaten for pain related to gout and can be combined with folic acid and plantain (another lawn weed).

Cinnamon: The oil or ground bark can be used as a compress to reduce pain. It has a natural warming affect that can sooth stiff and aching joints.

Comfrey: Helps speed up healing of bruised, sprained or fractured limbs. When used in a compress and applied to the area it can reduce the severity.

Cramp bark: As a known pain reducer cramp bark can be used with Prickly Ash and Wild Yam to relieve the pain in muscles.

Evening primrose oil: Take an infusion of Evening primrose root soaked in wine to reduce muscle strain and keep the blood flowing to muscle tissue.

Juniper: The crushed berries are used externally as a compress or poultice for sore and tired muscles.

Kava: The ground herb can be used in place of aspirin, acetaminophen and ibuprofen.

Parsley: Use parsley soaked in witch hazel to take the color out of bruises. Apply 2-3 times a day for about 1 hour each time.

Peppermint: The essential oil is used externally with *Eucalyptus and Lavender oil or
Rosemary. Simply place the combination of oils directly on the sore area or use with a carrier oil (baby oil works well with this.)

Rosemary: The oil in rosemary helps reduce muscle spasms. You can use this after a workout.

Sweet marjoram: The oil is used for muscle pain. This oil is gentle enough that it may be used on children.

Tea Tree Oil: First aid in a bottle, Tea tree oil can be used alone or with the above-mentioned oils.

Valerian: The stinky root of valerian is perfect for the gym, considering it already smells like an old sweat sock. Valerian eases muscle strain when used as a poultice.

Willow: The white willow bark can be chewed or brewed in a tea it is an aspirin like plant so if you are sensitive or allergic to aspirin you will not want to use willow bark.

Pre-sports rub

2 drops Rosemary oil
1 drop Lavender oil
1 drop Eucalyptus oil
Blend all oils and add 4 teaspoons of a base or carrier oil.
Apply this mixture to the body before exercising.

Post-sports rub

2 drops Lavender oil
1 drop Juniper oil
1 drop Rosemary oil
Mix oils together with 4 teaspoons of base oil and apply to the
body after exercise.

Stressed muscles with pain

3 drops Lavender
2 drops petit grain
1-2 drops Frankincense

Mix oils together and use in a warm bath. Soak until water becomes cool.

This may also be used as a rub by mixing oils together and using 2 drops of the mix per ounce of carrier oil.

Toothache

If you get a toothache it may be a sign that something else is going wrong. Infections and bacteria from damaged or diseased teeth can slip into the blood stream and cause more serious illnesses. If you have a toothache a temporary remedy will be okay but only use it long enough to get to a dentist to find out what the real problem might be.

Allspice: The oil of allspice can be used to calm a toothache, but do not swallow it. Also be careful that the oil is used only on the tooth and not the gum tissue around it because it may irritate the tissue and cause further discomfort

Bay: Use in toothpaste to help prevent tooth decay.

Bayberry: A decoction of bayberry can be used as a gum wash.

Caraway: For gingivitis use caraway with sage, peppermint, chamomile tincture, Echinacea, myrrh tincture, and clove oil.

Cayenne: You can make a poultice or compress with cayenne and apply to the tooth to confuse the pain. Be careful not to get it on your gums though.

Clove: The oil can be applied directly to the tooth or you can bite down on a whole clove and hold it. This will not only numb the pain but it will fight off any infections that may be there too.

Echinacea: Make a tea with Echinacea and use it as a mouthwash.

Ginger: Used with Red Pepper as a compress (caution very hot) —make into a paste and dip a piece of cotton. Place on tooth. (Be careful not to touch gums with paste).

Lemon: Eating lemons aids in the prevention of gingivitis. Use lemon juice as a gargle.

Myrrh: Great for treating mouth ulcers use with Echinacea as a mouthwash.

Peppermint: Use the flavored oil or chew fresh leaves to help with gum irritation.

Raspberry: A tea used as a mouthwash is used for bleeding gums.

Sage: Use in a gargle for inflammations of the mouth.

Sesame seed: Theses tiny little seeds are very useful for treating toothaches. Use sesame seed decoction on the tooth where pain is present.

Willow: The bark can be chewed or made into a tea or tincture. It works just like aspirin but also carries the same sensitivity warnings.

Skin

The skin is the first line of defense as well as the first thing people notice when they see us. Our skin has our history written all over it, how much time we spend in the sun, how old we are, what kind of day we have had our skin tells all. There is no wonder we spend millions of dollars just to improve the condition of our skin. But keeping the skin healthy does not have to cost a fortune, a little time and preparation can keep you looking your best without taking its toll on your budget.

Acne

It is well known that when you look good you feel good. These annoying blemishes can show up anytime and not just during adolescence. They can signify a number of different changes including hormone shifts and stress. Whether you suffer from the occasional ill-timed pimple, persistent blackheads, or chronic cases of acne these remedies can help. Some are for use externally on the blemishes themselves and others work internally to help keep it under control from the inside out. These remedies can be used alone or in combination with other treatments. For example your breakout may be caused by stress so you might treat the blemish on the outside while working on the stress from the inside.

Alfalfa: The use of alfalfa as part of a balanced diet can work wonders on all parts of the body including the promotion of healthy new skin cells. Alfalfa works from the inside out generating all around good health. It is easiest to add the sprouts to your meals or you can dry and powder the herb and place it inside capsules. You can also be creative and find other ways to take it.

Aloe Vera: A natural wonder, and a beautiful and useful addition to the home. This incredibly resilient plant is a living first aid kit. The small pieces of the plant can be broke off and the gel inside applied to the blemishes.

Calendula: Also known as pot marigolds, these plants are more than pretty, they are useful and edible. The bright orange flowers may be used as a tea to wash the face or other affected   areas. This treatment may be substituted with burdock and used in the same way. Calendula may also be used to make creams; it stimulates new skin cell growth and has anti-inflammatory properties.

Chamomile: A cup of this tea works wonders after a stressful day, but it can work just as well on your blemishes. Simply brew this tea as you normally would, then apply it to the affected areas with a clean cloth. It can also be used as a skin cream.

Dandelion: This pesky weed grows everywhere. Instead of trying to eliminate it from your yard, use it as a gift. It is a natural purifier. Dandelion leaves can be used in a salad. As well the flowers, leaves and dried roots can be used in teas. For leaves and roots use 2 teaspoons per 1 cup boiling water. The flowers can be used fresh by steeping 4-5 flowers in 1 cup hot water for about 5 minutes.

Garlic: Smelly but effective. Garlic cloves are very acidic and are a natural killer for the bacteria in the skin that can cause breakouts. Take one garlic clove and slice it open. Rub the sliced clove over the blemished area.

Lavender: This one smells better. Lavender is very soothing to the skin, and is especially useful if the outbreak is caused by stress. Use 1 part lavender oil to 10 parts rosewater or witch hazel as a wash. A few drops of the straight essential oil can be applied directly to the blemish.

Tea tree: Tea tree oil is a cure all kill all, it is safe and effective and may be used just like lavender oil but doesn't smell as pleasant. It has a very medicinal smell but I suppose for the guys that beats smelling flowery. Use 1 part tea tree oil to 10 parts rosewater or witch hazel as a wash.

Red clover: Use with Yellow Dock and Nettle to make a steam treatment for face and skin. Mix 1 part fresh or 2 parts dried herbs with boiling water. Place in a bowl or pan. Cover your head and the bowl with a towel and let the steam rise to your face for 3 to 5 minutes. You may also use as a wash. Mix 1 part fresh or 2 parts dried herb with warm water and infuse. Strain the herbs and use the water on the affected areas.

Rosemary: The oil from the rosemary plant can help treat acne for people with dry skin. The oil in the rosemary plant helps the skin produce its own natural oils.

Witch hazel: This can be found in the health and beauty aisle of your local store next to the alcohol. It can be used as an astringent and applied with cotton balls.

Acne drink

2 oz beet juice
2 oz celery juice
2 oz tomato juice
Mix well and drink 2-3 times daily.

Acne tea

Witch grass root
Elecampane root
*Juniper berries
Ground ivy
Elder leaves & flowers
Mix equal parts and steep 1 teaspoon of mixture in ½ cup boiling water,
Drink ½ to 1 cup unsweetened per day.

Mix celery seed with carrot juice as a cleansing drink.

Athlete's foot

When feet come in contact with fungus and are then

kept warm and damp, like in sweaty socks and shoes, Athlete's foot will result. The burning, itchy discomfort of athlete's foot can be eliminated and reoccurrences halted with treatment. Prevent athlete's foot by drying feet thoroughly, especially between the toes. Always wear clean socks and alternate shoes if possible. Also by wearing shower shoes or flip-flops when visiting pools, spas, gyms and other public wash areas you can reduce the chances of exposure to the fungus.

Alfalfa: By soaking feet in the warm reduced water of alfalfa it helps to kill the fungus. This is also good for tired feet. Eating alfalfa can fight fungal infections from the   inside.

Aloe Vera: Aloe gel can be applied directly on affected area to cool the burning and lessen the chances of infection due to cracked skin or open blisters. Let your feet   dry   before putting on fresh clean socks.

Cinnamon: Ground cinnamon mixed with equal parts cornstarch can be applied to affected area as a foot powder. This also works to deodorize shoes. Cinnamon oil may be applied directly to the foot. If skin irritation occurs dilute with 2 parts carrier oil.

Lemongrass: The crushed fresh herb has Antifungal properties and can be rubbed on affected areas. The fresh oils may cause skin irritation.

Red Clover: An infusion of the sweet little flower can be mixed with cornstarch to form a paste that is useful in treating athlete's foot.

Tea Tree Oil: Anything that can kill fungus is useful in treating athlete's foot. Tea tree oil is one of the most powerful kill all treatments on the market. It not only kills fungus but it kills the bacteria that can cause foot odor as well. Just use a few drops of Tea tree oil with a drop or two of Lavender oil directly on affected area or use in a foot wash.

Sprinkle cornstarch or baking soda in shoes when you are not wearing them to help absorb moisture and odor.

Anti-fungal oil

1 clove of garlic (chopped)
1 tablespoon ground cinnamon
1 teaspoon ground ginger
1 teaspoon chamomile
10 drops tea tree oil

Over low heat combine garlic, cinnamon, ginger and Chamomile with ½ cup safflower oil. Let simmer for 10-15 minutes. Strain through a cheese cloth and add tea tree oil. Cove immediately and allow it to cool before use.

Anti-fungal sauce

1 jar tomato sauce
1 tablespoon fennel
1 tablespoon dill
1 teaspoon basil
½ teaspoon celery salt
1-2 cloves of garlic
6 juniper berries

Combine all ingredients and simmer over low heat. Add to pasta.

Burns

As long as there is heat there will always be burns. But for as many types of burns including mild burns, scalds, sunburns, and steam injuries there are a number of ways to treat them.

These remedies are not for use with large area 2nd degree burns or 3rd degree burns of any size without the assistance of a doctor. Never put grease or ice directly on a burn. Always rinse area with cool water prior to treatment.

Alfalfa: Mash up some alfalfa sprouts and dip them in cold water to use as a cold compress or poultice and apply to the affected area.

Aloe Vera: Use the gel or a piece of the fresh plant applied directly to the area. Use of the plant is best for small areas as it may take too much of the plant to treat a very large burn.

Basil: The fresh leaves of sweet basil can be mashed applied to a burn to help it cool and heal.
8 fresh sweet basil leaves
1/8 tsp apricot kernel oil
Sterile cotton gauze
Surgical tape
Rinse leaves under cool water and pat dry and mince. In a small bowl combine basil and apricot oil and mash into a paste. Spread the paste on the gauze and cover burn for 2 hours securing it with the surgical tape. This may be repeated as necessary.

Blackberry: Fresh leaves can be dipped in cool spring water and laid loosely over the burned area. They can also be mashed and used in a poultice in the same way as   sweet   basil leaves.

Calendula: Make an ointment of these ordinary flowers to treat a number of skin ailment including burns.

Lavender oil: Place 4 drop in a bowl of cool water and gently wash the area. Apply 1 to 2 drops directly on the burn and let set. This helps to reduce the pain and heat of the burn as well as calm the nerves after the incident. It also feels good on fresh sunburns. Just rub a few drops gently into the sunburn.

St. John's Wort: You can make a lotion from the herb and apply to affected area. St. John's Wort is especially useful in the treatment of sunburns.

Yarrow: Particularly white yarrow can be used as an infusion to cool and heal burns.

Insects

From the nasty little pests of summer to the sneaky little hitchhikers the kids bring home, insects can interfere with your day no matter how hard you try to keep them out. Since some remedies can take a little while to make, (tinctures can take up to 2 weeks) and bug bites itch now, it is best to begin preparing for them a few weeks before spring.

Anise: The oil is used externally to kill lice and scabies.

Basil: Use tinctures or in lotions and creams to treat bites or just rub the area with leaves to reduce itching and inflammation. An ointment of basil works well on itchy bites and only takes a few minutes to prepare. The fresh crushed leaves can be rubbed on the skin as an insect repellant.

Pennyroyal: The oil or tincture of pennyroyal can be used as an insect repellant. Place it in a spray bottle for easy use.

Bayberry: Also known as waxberry for its use in candle-making, the leaves and berries can be used in ointments for relief of insect bites. Use topically.

Calamus: Can be used as a tincture for the treatment of lice and scabies. Apply it right on the affected area and allow it to sit for a while before washing it out.

Calendula: Use the fresh plant on a wasp sting.

Cinnamon: Use the oil to treat bee stings.

Echinacea: When taken in combination with golden seal and vitamins C and E, Echinacea helps bites heal faster. Echinacea tea can soothe the itch and inflammation when applied directly to the bite. Combine with eucalyptus for a cooling relief.

Lavender: Using the essential oil directly on the bites relieves the itching and discomfort and also helps them to heal faster.

Lemongrass: Use the fresh crushed herbs rubbed on skin for an insect repellant.

Insect repellant #1

1 part dried Rosemary
1 part dried Wormwood
1 part dried Lavender
1 part dried Sage
1 part dried Mint
Place all ingredients in a jar and cover with vinegar.
Let stand for 7 days. Use on clothing and exposed skin.

Insect repellant #2

4 oz Aloe Vera gel
4 oz light skin lotion
2 drams Citronella oil
½ dram Eucalyptus oil
½ dram Patchouli oil
Mix in a bottle and shake well
Do not use on face

Insect bites

1 teaspoon dried chickweed or one handful fresh made into tea and drunk 3 times a day. This mixture can also be used on skin to stop itching.

Skin injuries

The skin is the first line of defense against any illness or infection. Keeping the skin in good shape not only helps us look better, but also can prevent us from getting many illnesses. For scrapes, minor cuts, or other skin irritations there are many things that can be used to soothe and help heal. It is handy to keep some of these with you in your first aid kit just in case you need them.

Aloe Vera: The gel or a piece of the plant can be applied directly to the skin.

Bayberry: This great smelling berry can be used topically as a cream or lotion.

Benzoin: The tincture is used on cuts and scrapes to seal them and stop bleeding as well as fight off infections.

Castor: Finally a use for castor oils that you don't have to swallow. Castor oil can be used directly on cuts and scrapes.

Calendula: Use in a cream to treat minor cuts and scrapes. It helps to generate new skin cells and aids in reducing inflammation. The tincture helps relieve eczema.

Chamomile: Use a cream of chamomile to treat itch sore skin.

Echinacea: This can be used externally as a lotion or boiled in a tea and used to promote healing as well as fight off infection. The tea can be used internally or externally.

Elder: The flowers can be mixed with vinegar to make a healing ointment for skin problems.

Eucalyptus: The cooling oil is used externally to clean abrasions and sooth skin.

Evening primrose oil: This may be used with carrier oil for eczema and psoriasis and can also be taken internally to prevent these conditions.

Flax: The seeds can be used in a poultice to treat boils.

Lavender: Use 4 drops of lavender oil in water to clean the area plus one drop directly on the area to help heal and soothe it.

Lemongrass: Use as a tea to treat the symptoms of shingles. Use 2-3 leaf stalks (remove any damaged or icky spots) cut off bottoms about 6 inches up. Simmer in water for about 20 minutes then strain to remove the solids. The tea may be served hot or cold and can be kept for up to 24 hours in the refrigerator.

Mullein: Used for stings and scrapes, the crushed leaves can be made into a poultice.

Nettle: Without the stingers nettle can be used with Figwort and Burdock to make a cream for eczema. The stingers will cause skin irritation.

Peppermint: Use in creams and lotions to soothe irritated skin.

Red clover: Use the flowers as a compress to treat skin rashes.

Saffron: To make a soothing skin paste use powdered saffron and enough water to make it pasty then apply liberally to the affected areas. This paste is also a good way to   f i g h t the appearance of aging.

Sarsaparilla: When used for psoriasis, sarsaparilla can be combined with Burdock, Yellow Dock and Cleavers.

Sweet Marjoram: Use of sweet marjoram oil reduces signs of aging.

Tea Tree oil: This is an all purpose treatment for cuts, scrapes, scratches and bites.

Tea: Any kind of tea will do. If you have a few tea bags with you at all times just add a little water to them and you have a ready made poultice for most any type of skin   injury.

Yarrow: Use as a wash for treating cuts and wounds.

Psoriasis relief

1 anise bulk cut into pieces
3 cups of water
1 tablespoons basil
1 tablespoons parsley
1 cup steeped black tea

In a blender mix the anise until smooth. In small sauce pan heat water basil and parsley until boiling, reduce heat and simmer 45 min. Remove from heat and cool. Mix the resulting liquid with the anise and tea in small bowl (removing the herbs is optional). Apply mixture with clean cloth to area ever 30 min for 2 hours. Makes 2 cups will keep for 5 days if covered and refrigerated use every night as needed.

Warts

This section is proof that witches don't have warts, mainly because if they did they would have used one of these remedies to get rid of them. Warts are a type of virus that just about any one can get whether they have handled a toad or not. You could go to the doctor's office and have the unsightly blemish removed but that can be costly and painful. The natural way may of course take longer, most treatments require daily applications for a few weeks, but it is painless and more importantly more cost effective.

Aloe Vera: Break off a piece of the plant and apply it directly to wart.

Carob: Can used in a compress or poultice and placed on the wart.

Dandelion: Apply the fresh juice (the milky white stuff) of this common yard weed to the wart several times a day. (How is that for inexpensive?)

Garlic: Apply a clove of sliced garlic to the wart and cover with a bandage.

Lemongrass: The oils can irritate a wart right off the skin. Use caution though, it can also irritate unaffected skin.

Tea Tree Oil: Applied 3 to 4 times a day to wart. This may be alternated with cinnamon oil every other time.

Wounds

Much like the other skin injuries, wounds are subject to infection if not promptly treated. Wounds differ from scrapes and scratches in that they tend to be deeper, larger, and more serious. If the wound is very deep or become red and feverish, seek a doctor as soon as possible. Never poke anything into a wound and always wash the area thoroughly before treating to remove any debris.

Benzoin: The sticky gum tincture can be applied to the wound. This seals it and prevents infection.

Chamomile: The tea is used externally for treatment of wounds and to prevent infection.

Cinnamon: Ground cinnamon powder can be applied directly to the wound as an anti-bacterial agent. Caution, this may cause skin irritation.

Echinacea: Can be taken internally and used externally as a poultice.

Elder: Use the fresh cleaned leaves. These are bound externally to the wound.

Eucalyptus: Use the oil externally to clean the wound.

Garlic: Can be placed on a bandage that has been coated with castor oil and then placed over a wound. The garlic is very acidic so use only on a scabbed over wound due   t   o stinging.

Honey: Can be used on a dressing pad, change 1 to 3 times daily for the first few days; later you may change it every couple of days. Cover with a secondary dressing to   prevent   the honey form oozing.

Lavender: Wash the area with lavender oil and water to reduce pain and stress.

St. John's Wort: Can be used as an antiseptic lotion.

Safflower: A tincture of safflower may be used to treat wounds.

Tea Tree Oil: This wonderful medicinal oil can be used as an all purpose ointment.

Thyme: Can be used externally as a lotion.

Stomach

Overeating, the flu, motion sickness, gas, ulcers, cramp whatever the ailment if it has to do with the stomach it become of the center of our attention. When dealing with an upset stomach what ever the cause may be there are few things more important at the time. Listed here are some of the more common stomach ailments and some quick easy ways to treat them that will have you back on your feet in no time.

Diarrhea

There are many reasons we experience cases of diarrhea, foods and illnesses among them. The main concern with any diarrhea strike is of course dehydration and the loss of electrolytes. Lots of water and herbal teas can help prevent dehydration and sometimes put an end to the cause.

Apples: Eating the apple peel can stop diarrhea, but apple juice can increase it.

Bayberry: Drink in a tea to relieve diarrhea. Bayberry decoctions and tinctures are also helpful. For decoctions boil 1 teaspoon of powdered root bark in 1 pint of water   for 10-15 minutes. Add a bit of milk and drink cool 2 times a day. The decoction is bitter so you may want to take the tincture (1/2 teaspoon) 2 times a day.

Blackberry: A tincture of blackberry root can ease diarrhea. For use with infants mix 1 teaspoon of tincture with ½ cup warm water and take ¼ teaspoon every hour as needed. This can be substituted with raspberry leaves or use them together.

Carrots: Making carrot soup can stop diarrhea as well as nourish the body. It has been shown to reduce E. coli too.

Castor oil: One of the remedies handed down by grandmothers. A spoonful of castor oil taken as a tonic can stop diarrhea if you can get it swallowed.

Catnip: Easier and better tasting than a spoonful of castor oil, drink catnip tea to relieve diarrhea. Catnip is also useful for irritable children.

Garlic: Helps to kill off all kinds of bacteria. Add a clove or two to the carrot soup or other recipes. You can also crush the garlic cloves and place them in capsules if   you don't like the flavor.

Raspberry: The leaves brewed in a tea can ease diarrhea, while the fruit in large doses can cause it.

Diarrhea Tea #1

Oak bark
Horse chestnut bark
Mix 2 teaspoons per ½ cup water and drink unsweetened

Diarrhea Tea #2

1 part raspberry leaves
1 part mullein
1 part fenugreek
1 part St. John's Wort
1 part nettles

1 part ginger
1 part peppermint
Pour 4 cups of hot water over the herbs and let steep for
10 minutes to make a strong tea. Strain and drink 3-4 cups
a day. For extreme cases such as Montezuma you may add
the following: white willow bark powder, blue coshosh, blue
vervain, and valerian.

Aromatherapy massage

5 drops lavender
5drops patchouli
5 drops cypress
Mix in 20 ml of carrier oil and massage into abdomen.

Digestion

Sometimes what we eat doesn't always agree with us. Other
times it agrees so well that we indulge a little too much. Then
there is the times when no matter what we eat our stomachs
are just upset. This last case could be caused by any number of
other things including stress and fatigue. When digestion is at
its worst we need to get it back on track in order to maintain a
proper healthy balance.

Apple cider vinegar: Drink a glass of apple cider vinegar
mixed with water before meals to aid in digestion or take a
teaspoonful before or after the meal.

Allspice: The oil of allspice can be used to aid in digestion.
Use diluted due to irritation. Never take allspice oil in a
concentrated from.

Catnip: After dinner or a large meal, drinking catnip in a tea
can aid in digestion.

Catnip snacks

Dip fresh catnip leaves in egg whites and lemon juice then dust lightly with sugar and let dry. Enjoy as a healthy treat anytime.

Cinnamon: 1 to 2 drops of cinnamon oil added to tea or water will aid in digestive upset.

Clove: Can be added to foods to help with digestion.

Fennel: This sweet licorice flavored seed can be used in teas.

Ginger: Eat a bit of ginger before a meal to aid in its digestion.

Grapefruit: Eating a ½ of grapefruit or drinking a small glass of the juice can help settle indigestion.

Hops: Taken in capsules it stimulates the appetite and aids in digestion.

Lavender: Use an infusion for digestive problems.

Lemon: Sucking on a lemon wedge helps reduce stomach acid much like grapefruit.

Linden: The linden flower can aid in digestion when you drink the tea after dinner.

Peppermint: Use as a tea, extract or in capsule or chew on fresh leaves. Mint helps to settle the stomach after a meal. It makes a great breath freshener too.

Red Pepper: Use in place of black pepper, which can irritate the digestive tract. Red pepper is much healthier (not to mention spicier) and promotes better digestion.

Rosemary: Used as tea, rosemary is great for digestion.

Safflower: Can be added to food as well as being made in to a tea. Try cooking in safflower oil instead of lard or bacon grease.

Saffron: Its soothing actions go beyond the skin. Saffron can be made into a tea or added your favorite recipes to soothe digestion as well.

Sweet Marjoram: Use 1-2 teaspoons of the dried herb and flower per 1 cup of boiling water. Steep for 10 minutes and drink 3 times per day. If the taste doesn't suit you try mixing it with chicken or vegetable broth.

Flatulence (gas)

Aside from the bloating, cramping and discomfort of gas an ill timed attack can be embarrassing. Preventing the build up of gas is the key to stopping it from putting you under pressure.

Allspice: A kind of sweet kind of spicy berry that seems to form its flavor to what ever you add it to, allspice also has a flavor all its own. You can add 2-3 drops of allspice oil to sugar or a teaspoon of water.

Angelica: Either drink an infusion of angelica root or chew on the sweet angelica stems.

Angelica gas tea

1 pint boiling water
Pour over 1 ounce of bruised root or 10-30 grains powdered root.

Anise: If you like the taste of licorice (candy not the root) you can drink a tea made from crushed anise seeds.

Basil: Drink a tea made from the leaves helps to relieve gas. You could also use this in a broth but it might not work as well for gas relief.

Chamomile: Drink chamomile tea alone or with 1 drop cinnamon oil.

Fennel: Take 1 cup of a fennel infusion ½ hour before meals or 1-2ml of fennel tincture 3 times a day.

Ginger: When eaten or infused ginger helps to relieve gas and bloating.

*Lavende*r: Use the lovely blooms in a tea to relieve gas and bloating.

Peppermint: Ever wonder why you are served a mint after dinner? It's not just your breath. The leaves can be chewed, or brewed as a tea to aid in digestion and prevent pressure and bloating of gas build up. That sprig of parsley on your plate works the same way.

Sweet Marjoram: Similar to basil sweet marjoram can be used in a tea to ease flatulence.

Laxative

Sometimes our diet or the lack of discipline in it can cause our bodies to revolt. When all systems shut down and the body goes on strike, nothing will come out right. This can put us in a very uncomfortable state.

Aloe Vera: When taken internally Aloe Vera is a very strong laxative. Try it as a refreshing juice drink.

Basil: When used as a laxative you will want to use basil as a tea. Adding it to foods may increase complications especially if you are already bound up. It is best to take in   as many liquids as you can to get the juices flowing again.

Bladderwrack: A member of the Kelp family, Bladderwrack works like bran flakes. It can be found in most seafood stored of fish markets and used like lettuce on a sandwich or in a salad.

Celery seed: Can be eaten or used in tea. A little bit of the flavor can go a long way so you may want to add it a little at a time so it does not become over powering in food. In teas take by the teaspoonful several times a day.

Flax: When eaten the seeds act as a bulk laxative. Add some crushed seeds to your diet daily for regularity.

Safflower: The seeds or safflower tea is used as a laxative for adults but may be too powerful to be used by children.

Laxative drink

2 parts Tomato juice
1 part Sauerkraut juice
Mix well and drink

Laxative tea

Angelica
Alder buckthorn bark
Make into a tea and drink ½ to 1 cup daily (unsweetened) in
mouthful doses.

Nausea

Morning sickness, motion sickness, stress or just general nausea, which ever case and for what ever reason, it is one of the worst feelings in the world. There are a lot of known and unknown reasons for being nauseous, but what ever the reason here are a few ways to keep your stomach from flipping over and your wallet from flipping out.

Castor oil: It's that age old remedy again. It's not very yummy but if taken internally Castor oil is a good treatment for nausea when it is related to food poisoning.

Catnip: A little tastier than the castor oil, catnip tea will help settle your stomachs.

Cinnamon oil: Just 1 drop is added to a full glass of water or a cup of chamomile tea.

Clove: Drink the tea to alleviate altitude sickness.

Fennel: Chewing on a small handful of seed while traveling can settle stomachs and prevent motion sickness. Fennel can also be use in teas or tinctures for the same reason.

Ginger: Dinking 1 to 3 cups of ginger tea can calm the stomach spasms that tend to come with nausea. It helps stop the nausea, upset stomach and motion sickness as well.

Peppermint: The tea or a few fresh leaves can ease stomach irritation and settle nausea. If you have heartburn or acid reflux disease you may want to try something a little gentler though as peppermint can cause upsets in those areas.

Stomach ache

For the occasional tummy ache use these remedies alone or in conjunction with the remedies for nausea to soothe an irritated stomach.

Allspice: This sweet savory spice can be eaten with food or you can drink it as a tea.

Basil: Drink as a tea or broth as well as using it in foods.

Chamomile: Drinking this tea will help soothe your nerves as well as your tummy. Use chamomile as an ulcer protection tea.

Licorice: Use the root not the candy. Licorice can be chewed or used in a tea.

Red clover: Taken as a tea to help relieve pain of ulcers.

Saffron: When used in tea saffron can be very soothing on the stomach. You can also use saffron in many recipes.

Women

Today women face many issues PMS being only one of them. Fertility, sex drive, work, stress, family, it can all pile up quickly. But when women don't take time to focus on the issues of their bodies the little everyday stresses can turn into a major health problem. This section includes some of the more ailments that women face daily. Use these remedies with treatments for stress and anxiety. Also take a little time each day to appreciate and pamper yourself or the woman in you life. She is a goddess.

Cramps (pms)

When it is that time of the month nothing feels worse than menstrual cramp. With the combination of bloating, fatigue, headache, cramps, and the flux in hormones it is no wonder women get irritable. Keeping yourself balanced is easy if you can first make yourself comfortable. It is always important for women to stay focused in order to stay healthy but it is most important during this powerful time of the month.

Allspice: For cramps use allspice as a tea. If they are severe you can make a poultice from the crushed berries. Allspice can be irritating to the skin so be sure to use a cloth. It is wonderful when added to food.

Caraway: Use caraway oil in a compress or a bath to relieve symptoms of PMS.

Cat's claw: Cat's claw has been shown in new research to have many uses in pain control. The herb can be used as a tea, tincture or in capsules for the management of pain and discomfort.

Chamomile: A wonderful tea for moods associated with PMS. The oil can also be rubbed on the painful areas to sooth away cramps. Place a cloth filled with chamomile flowers under the faucet while running a warm bath.

Cramp bark: Drink a tea made from cramp bark or use as a compress for cramps.

Dong quai: May be used alone or added to any tea to help relieve pain. The foliage can be eaten like celery as well as the flower bud, which can be added raw to salads or cooked and eaten. The young shoots are sometimes candied and used as a treat or to decorate desserts.

Evening primrose oil: Excellent when rubbed over affected area, use with a carrier oil, or it can be taken internally. The benefits from EPO may take several cycles to begin working but it is well worth the wait if you suffer from server cramps.

Feverfew: This can be chewed or used in teas as well as taken in capsules to reduce symptoms of PMS. Some times mouth irritation can occur when feverfew is chewed. If you experience discomfort or if mouth sores develop, use less frequently or brew as a tea.

Raspberry: The leaves used in a tea drank several times a day as needed reduces pain and promotes uterine health. I would recommend begin drinking this tea 2-3 days prior to the onset of your period as well as through the duration. This is a great tea hot or cold.

Skullcap: You can add skullcap to any tea to ease the tension associated with PMS. Try it mixed with valerian and chamomile just before bedtime.

Sweet Marjoram: Used in a tea sweet marjoram can encourage sluggish menstruation and ease cramps.

Squaw vine: Also known as squaw berry has been used by American Indians for centuries to aid in female health. It promotes uterine health as well as aid in relief of irregular menstruation and cramps.

Cramp tea

2 parts Raspberry leaves
2 parts Catnip
1 part Squaw vine
1 part Cramp bark
1 part Black Cohosh
Make into a tincture and take 1 drop per 10 lbs body weight.
Can be used as a tea by steeping catnip and raspberry
Simmer all other ingredients then mix well.

Menstruation

Aside from the cramping and discomfort of your period, there are sometimes other issues to deal with. Sometimes the flow can be too heavy or sometimes it can be sluggish. Then there are things such as menopause that can cause just as much discomfort as the periods themselves. The following remedies can be used alone or in co-operation with the remedies in other areas.

Alfalfa: The leaves in a tea will help with the symptoms of menopause.

Angelica: The seeds of Angelica promote menstruation. They can be lightly roasted and eaten as a treat or placed on salads. Angelica is one of the most useful and visually appealing flowers we can grow.

Bayberry: You can use bayberry in a tea, decoction or tincture taken for menstrual symptoms.

Black cohosh: Works in the body like estrogen to help relieve menopause symptoms.

Cramp bark: Handy to have for all sorts of menstruation problems, cramp bark is also used for excessive bleeding and menopause. It can be used alone or with Black Haw and Valerian.

Dong quai: You can take Dong quai to regulate your hormones and aid with the symptoms of menopause.

Evening Primrose oil: Over time 2-3 grams of oil taken daily can reduce the symptoms of menstruation and menopause.

Feverfew: As well as a pain reliever feverfew is used as a treatment for sluggish menstrual flow. Chew up to 2 leave a day unless irritation occurs then use less or try it in a different form.

Mugwort: Used in a tea it helps to ease heavy menstrual flow.

Saffron: The soothing yellow saffron helps to regulate menstrual disorders.

Skullcap: Brewed with other PMS or related teas, skullcap helps with tension and irritability.

St. John's Wort: Taken in capsules or brewed in tea St. John's wort is used to treat stress due to menopause.

Soy: Taken regularly soy helps with symptoms of menopause including hot flashes.

Yarrow: As an infusion it helps to relieve cramps.

Menstrual problems

St. John's Wort
European mistletoe
Mix equal parts and parboil 1 teaspoon in ½ cup water,
Then steep covered for 5 minutes,
Take warm in mouthful doses.

Sex drive

Sometimes women find themselves in need of a little help to get the fires burning again. Many things can affect the sex drive, hormone balances, stress, diet or age can all by factors. Time and tenderness is always a good starting point but for those times when you just need a little more try adding some of these sexy little herbs to your day.

Anise: Drinking the seeds in a tea can help to increase the female sex drive.

Black cohosh: Taken in capsules or teas and infusions Black cohosh helps to balance the female hormone levels. It is also good for PMS

Chaste tree berry: This was once used to insure chastity in a lover but it also helps to promote sexual desire.

Dong Quai: Provides the body with a natural estrogen which can help during menopause and other times when estrogen levels begin to drop.

Licorice root: Another estrogen supplement that also reduces stress levels and increases energy.

Weight loss

Diet and weight loss has become a way of life for millions of people. It seems more and more people are coming up with new fad diets and weight loss programs not to mention the millions of dollar worth of exercise equipment. But obesity is still a major threat. Proper diet and regular exercise is fundamental for body and mind, but that does not mean spending thousands of dollars on low this high that diet whatever. A little self control and moderation can keep you happy and health.

Energy
If you are feeling run down or just need a boost there are healthier ways to achieve that than a candy bar and a cup of coffee. Many athletes have used these remedies to get an extra push while competing.

Calamus: Some cultures have chewed pieces of Calamus for increased endurance. If you choose to do this, I would suggest you use only a little bit and check for a reaction. If there is no reaction you may gradually increase the amount you use. The taste may take some time to acquire though so you may want to try brewing a tea or infusion.

Carob: Carob seeds can be roasted, ground and used as a substitute for coffee. This also works with cleaver, flaxseeds and for decaf use dandelion roots. Carob is also a great chocolate substitute.

Garlic: When eaten, garlic increases physical strength and energy. It is excellent for athletes.

Ginger: When you eat ginger you can increase your stamina.

Ginseng: Increases endurance. It is a mental and physical stimulant.

Green tea: When you drink green tea daily it gives you a refreshing steady energy.

Licorice: Helps to increase endurance and vitality.

Rosemary: A rosemary infusion used in bath wakes you up. Do not use before going to bed.

Sweet marjoram: Another good wake up herb. Use in eggs at breakfast or with rosemary in your morning bath.

Energy tea

1 part Juniper berry
2 parts blackberry leaves
5 parts wild strawberry leave
10 parts raspberry leaves
Steep 1 teaspoon in ½ cup hot water for 5-10 minutes,
Sweeten to taste.

Metabolism

One of the biggest parts of trying to lose weight is trying to get our metabolism back on track. It seems the older we get the slower it is. When our metabolism is functioning properly we are able to process the foods we eat before they can be stored in our system as fat. Once we speed up the metabolism process it is not uncommon for us to eat more. Metabolism is like a fire, the more we feed it the hotter it burns but first we must stoke to the fire to get it burning again.

Apple cider vinegar: As well as the other health benefits that come from drinking or taking apple cider vinegar a glass or two a day of apple cider vinegar and water increases the metabolism. It is one of the fastest ways to get the fires rolling.

Bladderwrack: Eating kelp helps speed up metabolism and is good source of calcium and other minerals. Use it on salads and sandwiches.

Yerba Mate: Used in teas to help boost the metabolism without Ephedra.

Metabolism tea #1

Juniper berry

Milfoil

Nettle

Mix equal parts in a tea use 1 teaspoon per ½ cup boiling water
Take ½ to 1 cup daily in mouthful doses, sweeten with honey

Metabolism tea #2

Juniper berry
Birch leaves
Chamomile

Mix equal parts in a tea use 1 teaspoon per ½ cup boiling water

Take ½ to 1 cup daily in mouthful doses, sweeten with honey
The other major problem with trying to lose weight is the
excess baggage otherwise known as cellulite. One way to get
rid of it is use the following oil massaged into the problem
areas.

Cellulite oil

5 drops fennel oil
4 drops rosemary oil
2 drops juniper oil
4 drops lavender oil
20 ml carrier oil
Massage gently into affected areas morning and night.

PART 4

A closer look

A

Alder buckthorn (Rhamus frangula) is a thornless bush or shrub with tiny green flowers that are followed by red berries. The berries turn black as they ripen.

Alfalfa (Medicago sativa) is a slender busy plant with small pale purplish colored flowers. The whole plant can be used for various different purposes but they are blandly flavored.

Allspice (Pimenta dioica) also known as Jamaica pepper is an evergreen tree identified by numerous small white flowers that are followed by the small reddish-brown berries. These berries have a mixed flavor that is reminiscent of nutmeg, clove, cinnamon and pepper.

Aloe Vera is a thick meaty plant. It almost resembles a leafless fern. Its sharp spindles can be broken off from the plant and used directly; the plant has the means to heal itself as well as us if it is used sparingly and given enough time to re-grow.

Althea (Althaea officinalis) See marshmallow

Angelica (Lamium album) also known as Archangel has a large thick stem with course leaves that grow along the length of it. It is covered with small white flowers that hang just below the leaves. All parts of this plant are eatable and sweet to the taste.

Anise (Pimpinella anisum) clusters of off white flowers on multi-branched stalks. This aromatic plant gives way to flavorful seeds that can be used in many ways both medicinally and in cooking.

Apple cider vinegar is usually found in grocery stores. This form of vinegar has more nutritional and healing properties than white or malt vinegar and can be used in much the same way.

Asparagus (Asparagus officinalis) the fleshy spears or shoots of this plant have been used for centuries for its medicinal properties. The plant sprouts white flowers that give way to red berries that can be harmful if eaten.

B

Banana fruit of the banana tree is not only a tropical delight it is a healthy choice for snacks and quick recipes. The banana peel is most notable yellow but some species can be red or brownish in color.

Basil (Ocimum basilicum) also known as sweet basil is part of a very large family. The herbs name is associated with the legendary basilisk, a giant deadly snake. The plant stalks are covered with a light hair and small clusters of pick flowers are seen at the base of the leaves.

Bay (Laurus nobilis) the leaves grow on a small tree or shrub and though commonly used only for flavor in foods, the bay leaf or laurel has played a significant role in magic.

Bayberry (Myrica pensylvanica) also called wax myrtle due to the wax that forms on the berries, which can be boiled down to make the fragrant bayberry candle. The nuts or leaves are suitable substitutions for the bay leaf.

Belladonna (Atropa bella-donna) also known as Deadly

nightshade was named for one of the Greek fates "Atropos" who cut the threads of life. Despite its poisonous nature, it has been widely used for medicinal purposes. The plant has beautiful purple blooms and produces black or deep purple berries that have a sweet flavor and have been responsible for the death of many children who have eaten them.

Benzoin (Styrax Benzoin) also known as gum Benjamin for its gummy resins that has been used for many treatments of respiratory ailments. The evergreen tree has gray bark that produces the resin and bright green leaves with a downy gray underside as well as white cup shaped flowers.

Bilberry (Vaccinium myrtillus) also known as huckleberry or European blueberry, have glossy green leaves and stems with bell shaped greenish pink flowers that give way to bluish black colored berries when ripe. It is a member of the same family as the cranberry that has dark green leaves and stems and pink bell shaped flowers that give way to reddish black colored berries when ripe.

Birch (Betula) there are many different species of birch and most all of them can be used medicinally as well as magically. The tree is identified by its white and silver peeling bark and its soft, droopy branches. Birch is used for wands and brooms as well as for healing.

Blackberry (Rubus fruticosus) the bramble of thorny vines or stems produce purple or deep reddish black berry. It is related to the raspberry as well as many different cross breeds such as loganberries and dewberries. The leaves and fruits are used for food and medicines.

Black cherry (Prunus serotina) part of the family of trees that include cherries, plums, peaches almond and apricots, the trees have been used in many culinary and medicinal ways. The tree has shiny narrow leaves and fragrant white flowers and produce small black or dark red berries. Both the fruit and bark of the tree are used. The juice of the cherry can be used as a substitute for blood in magic rituals.

Black Cohosh (Actaea racemosa) has a slender bottle brush spike on whish small unpleasant smelling white flowers bloom. Unlike blue cohosh, black cohosh is not given during pregnancy. This herb root is bitter so would best be taken in capsules.

Black walnut (Juglans nigra) because the tree bares such large leaves and nuts, it was named for the Latin "Jupiter" and "acorn". Its main medicinal use is digestive but the nut as well as the husk can also be beneficial for many other treatments.

Bladderwrack (Fucus vesiculosus) is one of many forms of marine algae. It is characterized with having air bladders to give the plant buoyancy. It is leathery greenish-brown seaweed that can be used to give food a salty sweet flavor. It was also beneficial in the discovery of iodine.

Blue Cohosh (Caulophyllum thalictroides) is also known as squaw root due to its multiple benefits to women's health and childbirth. The yellowish green to purple leaves have flowers that appear star shaped. Dark blue berries follow new leaves.

Bog bean (Menyanthes trifoliata) this plant is most commonly found near water thus the name bog. Its leaves shaped similar to the fava bean and it has white lacey flowers that are tinted pink on the outer side. The leaves can be dried and used in teas and are sometimes used as a substitute for hops when brewing beer.

Butchers broom (Ruscus aculeatus) a low growing shrub with extraordinarily large red berries this plant got its name from its use in sweeping out butcher's shops. It grows in small clumps with flat leaf like stems that have sharp tips.

The young shoots can be eaten much like asparagus as well as the entire plant can be used in medicine specifically as an anti-inflammatory.

Burdock (Arctium lappa) named for the burs that cling to animals and passers by the plants have large leaves and purplish thistle like flowers. The burdock is mostly responsible for the development of Velcro, which was designed after a scientist examined the way its hooked burs clung to the looped weaving of his clothes. Used medicinally in many ways the leaves, young shoots, stems and roots are also eatable.

C

Calamus (Acorus calamus) also called sweet flag or sweet sedge is a semi evergreen plant with a citrus fragrance. Its long flat leaves resemble the iris and produce small yellow green flowers on stems that resemble the leaves.

Calendula (Calendula Officinalis) also known as the pot marigold they are widely used to decorate gardens. This flowering weed has bushy leaves with branched stems and flowers in sunny arrays of golds and oranges. The petals can be used as a substitute for saffron and can also be added to many recipes including fresh salads.

Caraway (Carum carvi) this fern like plant has flat wide spread leaves that resemble fingers and small white or pink flowers that are arranged in clumps. It produces a 5 ribbed fruit that hold the widely used seeds. The leaves taste similar to parsley and the roots can be cooked and eaten as a vegetable. These are the seeds commonly seen in sauerkraut.

Castor (Ricinus communis) is a fast growing shrub that can sometimes grow to be as large as a tree. Its large palm like leaves sprout from dark red stems on long stalks. The female plant has yellow-green flowers with a red stigma that are followed by reddish brown seedpods, which contain the grayish brown tick shaped seeds. Even though all parts of this plant especially the seeds are toxic it has been used medicinally since the 1780's.

Catnip (Nepeta cataria) so named for its pleasurable effect on most cats, it has been used medicinally. The slightly hairy stems have a gray-green colored leaf and white flowers with purple spots that grow similar to clover. The mint flavor that gives it the name catmint is infused into teas or can be eaten in salads. The plant has a lemon scented relative that has no known medicinal use.

Cat's claw (Uncaria tomentosa) named for its claw like hooks it is becoming one of the most widely researched herb for the treatment of such ailments as arthritis, cancer and AIDS. Though it has been used in Peru for more than 2000 years it has only been used internationally since the 1980's. Since it has many interactions and contradictions with other treatments, use of cat's claw should be reserves for qualified practitioners.

Cayenne (Capsicum annuum) one of the many types of peppers it grows on branched stems with green or white flowers. It produces hollow bell, round or crescent shaped fruits that can vary in color. The cayenne is generally crescent shaped and may start out green or yellow and ripen to red. The fruit may cause irritation when handled which is one of the reasons it works well for pain and inflammation. The irritation allows more blood flow to the area and promotes healing.

Celery (Apium gravrolens) the wild form of the culinary delight (A. dulce) has a strong aroma with tiny green and white flowers that turn into the grayish brown seeds. Though wild celery has been used for centuries it is the milder domestic version that is recommended due to the flavor and toxicity of wild celery.

Chamomile (Anthemis tinctoria, Chamaemelum nobile, Matricaria recutita) there are many types of chamomile, each with specific uses. For dyes and colors the A. tinctoria with its bright yellow flowers was used in Turkey for rugs. It was later named C. nobile or Roman chamomile for its apple like aroma which is released when the flower is walked on making it a preferred choice for lawns, gardens and footpaths. M. Recutita or German chamomile is not as fragrant and has a more bitter taste than its Roman counter part but works just as well medicinally. All have a small daisy look with delicate white petals and yellow except for the A. tinctoria, which has golden yellow daisy like flowers with yellow centers.

Chickweed (Stellaria media) a small slender weed with white star shaped flowers it can endure even through the winter is some milder climates. Once used as a food for domestic birds it is useful medicinally for skin conditions and arthritic pain. Sprigs of chickweed can be added to salads, cooked as greens or liquefied with other herbs to make tonics.

Cinnamon (Cinnamomum Zeylanicum) grown as an evergreen tree it has thick leathery leaves and a papery bark that is cultivated for its sweet and warming properties and used in baking as well as medicine. The tree produces small white and yellow flowers that are followed by purple berries.

Citronella comes from a fragrant grass grown in South Asia. It is made into oil and used as a perfume or as insect repellents.

Cleavers (Galium aparine) a climbing bristly stem with small white flowers that are followed by greenish purple fruits. The entire plant including the seeds can be used medicinally many different ailments or eaten as a diet to promote weight loss. The seeds may be roasted like coffee.

Clove (Syzygium aromaticum) is the dried flower buds of an aromatic evergreen tree. The flowers have pink petals that fall off upon opening to reveal a yellow stamen that turns brown as it dries. They release their oils when squeezed.

Coltsfoot (Tussilago farfara) a robust creeping flower that grows best in the wild it has a large round heart shaped leaf and a dandelion like yellow flower. The young leaves, flowers and buds are used uncooked in salads as well as in soups, teas and wines.

Cornsilk (Zea mays) the female flower of the corn, which is separate from the male part, is high in potassium, which can be lost in urine due to the diuretic effect of the herb. The female flowers are in clusters in the leaves ending in the long filaments or cornsilks, and enclosed by the husk where they are followed by an ear of corn.

Cramp bark (Viburnum opulus) a semi-evergreen shrub or tree with 3 or 5 leaves and flat topped clusters surrounded by white flowers. It produces bright red round fruit that can cause mild stomach upset if eaten raw. The bark is peeled before the leaves change colors or open and used to make medication for use with menstrual problems.

Cranberry (Vaccinium macrocarpon) See Bilberry

D
Dandelion (Taraxacum officinale) this common lawn weed is identified by its jagged leaves and fluffy yellow blossom on a thick single stem. The yellow bloom turns puffy and white when the seeds are ready to spread. All parts of this plant are eatable in salads, teas medication and wine.

Devil's claw (Harpagophytum procumbens) used as mouse traps in Madagascar; this tuber grows in sandy dry areas and has many stems with large reddish purple flowers. It has been use by locals as a natural decoction.

Dill (Anethum graveolens) looks similar to fennel except it is more slender with a single stem and a flat rather than shiny look. The leaves smell like parsley and caraway and are gray-green in color. It supports flat clusters of yellow flowers that produce fragrant seeds, the smell of which can stop hiccups.

Dong quai (Angelica sinensis) a relative of Angelica archangelica, but not to be confused with Angelica (L. album) the A. sinensis version has many short purplish stems with flush segmented leaves and green flowers in clumps.

E

Echinacea there are many species that make up the Echinacea family most of which can be used interchangeably. It grows on a single stalk and is daisy like in appearance. The blooms can be white or purplish in color.

Elder (Sambucus nigra) or common elder is one of several trees, shrubs and flowers in this family. It is often called the "medicine chest" for its many medical uses. All parts are useful but modern uses are usually limited to the flowers. The large shrub has a gray-brown bark and the foliage has a foul smell when crushed. It bears tiny flat topped white clusters of flowers followed by round black berries. Do not eat the leaves or raw berries.

Elecampane (Inula helenium) thick stems and yellow flowers with sharp pointed leaves it resembles the daisy. The root can be used for medicines or candied as a treat.

Ephedra (Ephedra distachya) also known as Ma huang is a small evergreen shrub with tiny leaves. The male and female plants must be grown together to produce the red meaty fruits. This plant has been restricted in sales due to its speed like reaction but has previously been used medicinally for bronchial problems as well as by athletes. A second species of Ephedra (E. nervadesis) also called "Mormon tea" is less powerful and not typically used in medicine. It was named "Mormon tea" because it is used as a substitute for caffeine beverages prohibited by the Mormon faith.

Eucalyptus: there are over 600 species of this tree native to Australia. Each type of tree has a distinct sent and or use. The tree itself is among the largest growing trees in the world. (Eucalyptus globules) the species generally used for it vapor benefits in breathing treatments as well as in ointments for sports rubs.

Evening primrose (Oenothera biennis) a tall flowering plant that can thrive well in most soil conditions, its seeds are the source of Evening primrose oil (EPO). The evening primrose has a long thick stalk with many large leaves that encircle it from base to tip. It has large cup shaped flowers that open in the evening, thus its name. The seed pods are long and covered with fine hairs and are the source of the valuable oil. All parts of the evening primrose are eatable in a variety of ways both cooked and raw.

Eyebright (Euphrasia officinalis) the wild parasitic flower grows in grassy areas near a host plant. It has small round white flowers with purple veins and a centered yellow mark on tall leafy stems. The veins on the flowers where said to resemble the eye problems which they were used to treat such as blood shot eyes.

F

Fennel (Foeniculum vulgare) a bulbous clump with hollow stems and dull yellow flowers, it has a similar flavor and scent to anise. It has many uses for digestion as well as to aid in lactation but is most commonly used for its flavor in fish and liqueurs. All parts of fennel are eatable and fragrant and can be cooked or eaten raw in salads.

Fenugreek (Trigonella foenum-graecum) as aromatic plant

with 3 leaf clusters sprouting from a long stem, it produces one or two yellow-white flowers that have a hint of purple at the base. Used primarily as a spice, the leave and seeds are added to a number of recipes for both their flavor and their medicinal value.

Feverfew (Tanacetum parthenium) a member of the daisy family this short lived summer flower is a natural remedies for most types of headache including margarines. The species is made up of many forms from small white flowers that resemble the daisy, to large yellow puffy flowers. Some species of the flower offers a natural insecticide such as the T. cinerariifolium.

Flax seed (Linum) also known as linseed, it grows on upright narrow stems with dull green leaves and light blue flowers. The whole plant including the oil is beneficial for many remedies, but taken in excess can be fatal. Flaxseed oil may be taken as a substitute for EPO or the seed can be added to foods and ground and roasted as coffee.

G

Garlic (Allium sativum) the most pungent and beneficial of this family of bulbous plants, it has been used in flavoring foods as well as in medicines for centuries. The bulbs are usually clustered with 5-15 cloves per bulb covered in a white or pinkish papery skin. The bulb produces a long stalk with flat leaves and greenish white to pink flowers. Though generally only the bulb is used the young leaves, stalks and flowers have a milder taste.

Ginger (Asarum canadense) a wild woodland plant it is used as a ground cover in gardens for its creeping nature. Its use medicinally stems from it warming effect and is often combined with Ephedra for colds and fevers. It has a slender stalk from which it produces fuzzy heart shaped leaves that smell strongly of ginger. It also has purplish flowers that are grown at about ground level.

Ginseng (Panax ginseng) a carrot shaped root with branches it grows a long stalk with 5 leaves and small 5 petal flowers that are yellow-green in color. It produces red berries that contain two seeds each. A related but milder form of the species, (P.quinquefolius) known as American ginseng is generally given to children. It looks similar to the P. ginseng with the exception that the leaves grow in groups of 3-7 per stalk.

Goldenseal (Hydrastis canadensis) grows near the American ginseng; the bright yellow root produces a large palm like leaf with tiny clusters of green-white flowers. The flowers are replaced by a red berry that can not be eaten.

Ground ivy (Glechoma hederacea) a mint like lawn weed, it is grown as ground cover for many lawns and gardens. It was replaced by hops for its medicinal use as a cough treatment. It creeps with mostly evergreen leaves and tubular pink or bluish flowers. The whole plant can be used in teas or syrups for coughs and breathing difficulties.

H

Hawthorn (Crataegus laevigata) there are many species and hybrids of these densely branched shrubs. They have thorns and rounded leaves as well as fragrant white flowers that are followed by dark red berried. The flowers, leaves and berries are used mainly for circulatory and heart disorders. The hybrids can be used interchangeably with each other with the same result.

Hops (Humulus lupulus) a colorful climbing plant often used to make beer; it has been used as a sleep aid by Native Americans. The plant grows male and female parts on separate branches and it is the female that produces the hops under light green fragrant bracts. The male is a tiny green flower that grows in clusters on branches.

Horehound (Ballota nigra) named for its ability to repel livestock, is used mainly for garden borders. Its hairy pungently scented leaves are not as valued for its medicinal properties but the tubular purple flowers attract bees. The whole plant can be used in infusions, tinctures or as dried herbs for nausea, but its bitter taste makes capsules a preferred method of use.

Horse chestnut (Aesculus hippocastanum) named for its ability to treat choughs in horses the large tree produces sticky buds that give way to spikes of little white flowers. The nuts and twigs of the horse chestnut or Buck eye are poisonous.

J
Juniper (Juniperus communis) is a dark green or blue-green shrub with short pointy needles that have a white stripe on them. The berries are found only on the female plants, which grow separately from the male. The green berries ripen to black with a gray flower. Juniper can irritate the system so it is best used with corn or marshmallow.

K
Kava (Piper menthysticum) a robust evergreen shrub with thick meaty stems and rounded heart shaped leaves, this fragrant lilac scented plant is one of a thousand different species of pepper. It is the root rather than the berries that are used for its medicinal properties

Kelp (Laminaria) also known as seaweed. There are many different types of kelp most ranging from olive green to brownish in color. Kelp can be found along various coastlines at low tide usually anchored to rocks. Kelp can be used as a salt substitute as well as a bulk laxative and its many vitamins and minerals.

L
Lavender (Lavandula) there are many types of lavender hybrids grown for their oils, blooms and medicinal value.

Common to most lavender types are long thin stalks with thin upswept leaves and white, pink or purplish clusters of blooms on the top of the stalk giving it a bottle brush shape. Lavender is very soothing and is commonly used in teas and aroma therapy.

Lemons (Citrus limon) a small tree with narrow light green leaves and long sharp thorns, it has purple buds with white scented flowers that give way to large yellow fruits.

Lemon balm (Melissa officianalis) also known as Sweet Melissa is a lemon scented plant with large oval leaves and pale white or yellow flowers that form in clusters. A member of the mint family, the whole plant can be used mostly in teas but the fresh leaves add flavor to salads and vinegar dressings as well.

Lemongrass (Cymbopogon citrates) a large aromatic grass with a distinct lemony scent. Its large long blades can be used in many remedies but is mostly used for its oil. The neat oil of lemongrass can cause irritation to the skin.

Licorice (Glycyrrhiza glabra) the hardy root of the plant produces downy stems and many oval leaves on the same stem. The root is sweet and can be chewed like a piece of candy. The plant produces small blue or violet flowers in a lose bottle brush formation. Over use of this plant can lead to water retention and high blood pressure.

Linden (Tilia cordata) a large pale tree with light wood that can be made into musical instruments it has dark green heart shaped leaves. It hosts clusters of fuzzy yellow flowers that are followed by small round green fruits. The flowers can have a narcotic effect when mature, so it is best to use only the newly opened flowers for teas or infusions.

Lobelia (Lobelia inflata) also known as Indian tobacco or pukeweed the plant has been used for its narcotic qualities.

This downy shrub produces light blue with pink flowers and bright green leaves along the whole stem. The plant is one of the ingredients for anti-smoking tobaccos. As well over use of the plant can cause nausea and vomiting.

Lungwort (Pulmonaria officinalis) a clump forming plant with thick hairy stems and white spots on the leaves that are also hairy. It has funneled flowers that open pink then turn blue. The young leaves can be added to soups and salads as well as used in teas or syrups for coughs.

M

Marshmallow (Althaea officinalis) it is grown from a meaty tap root and forms a downy stem with soft fuzzy round or pointed leaves. A soft pink flower is produced in the center of the plant. The roots can be used as a substitute for egg whites or used in medicine making as well as candy. The leaves and flowers are also eatable and can be used for many bronchial ailments.

Milfoil (Achillea millefolium) See yarrow

Mint (Mentha) the name given to a collection of plant that carries the characteristic sweet, cooling aroma and sensation in their oils. Some mints can be hybridized to form unique flavors or aromas such as lemon mint or chocolate mint. Water mint has reddish purple stems with fuzzy leaves and lilac flowers. Its scent is similar to pennyroyal and peppermint. Pennyroyal is a thick clump of small round leaves and lilac flowers on thick stems that grow low to the ground. Peppermint is often a creeping purplish plant with jagged leaves and lilac-pink flowers on spikes.

Mistletoe (Viscum album), which grows on the upper branches of a host tree, is actually a parasite. It takes on the properties of the host tree and was collected by the Druids mostly or solely for the oak. It is an evergreen shrub with branched stems and yellow-green leaves that are leathery. It has clusters of yellow flowers followed by sticky white berries on the separate female plants. All parts of the plant but especially the berries are deadly if eaten. It is said that young Druids had to spend many years training in order to learn how the use the mistletoe in healing without killing the patient.

Motherwort (Leonurus cardiaca) has purple stems with flat leaves that resemble the maple leaf. Pink-white flowers with purple spots are produced along the shaft or stalk. The Chinese version of the plant has thin more deeply cut leaves. The whole plant is used medicinally for female problems as well as heart and nervous issues. The flowers can be used to flavor beers or soups as well as tea.

Mugwort (Artemisia) a family of herbs including southernwood, wormwood, tarragon, Mugwort, and absinthe these herbs are mostly bitter and pungent. Southernwood is a semi-evergreen shrub with grayish green leaves and tiny yellow flowers. Wormwood looks similar with long hairs on both sides and insignificant clusters of yellow flowers. Tarragon has branched stems and smooth leaves with small green licorice scented flowers. Absinthe is a tall upright stem with dull yellow flowers and grayish green leaves. Mugwort has purplish red stems and dark green leave with white an underside and small red-brown flowers.

Mullein (Verbascum thapsus) a hearty plant it has long bottle brush like spikes of 5 petaled yellow flowers. It has large towering flat leaves that are covered in a fine hair. The leaves and flowers have been used for respiratory complaints and the leaves have been smoked as a substitute for tobacco.

Myrrh (Commiphora myrrha) the resin from a collection of trees all having similar properties it has been used as a pain killer since biblical times, said to have been offered to Jesus prior to his death. It is a fragrant thorny shrub with thin fern like leaves and yellow-red flowers with 4 petals. The resin is collected and hardened for use and can be used to make the oils. The oils should not be taken internally.

N
Nettle (Urtica dioica) also known as stinging nettle due to its sharp hairs that sting and irritate the skin when touched.

It has creeping yellow roots and jagged pointy leaves that are covered in tell-tell stinging hairs. Small green flowers grow in clusters along the stems. The whole plant can be used medicinally and the young leaves can be cooked as greens or made into soups. It is not recommended to eat uncooked leaves.

O
Oat (Avena sativa) a tall grass with flat leaves, its seeds are pale yellow or golden in color. The seeds and the stalk or straw can be used. It contains important oils as well as protein and vitamin E and is good for your heart, skin and nervous system

Olive (Olea europaea) an evergreen tree with gray bark and gray-green leathery leaves with a silver rough underside, it is one of the oldest known trees reaching over 1000 years old in some areas. Its cream color flowers give way to oval green fruits that ripen to black. Green unripe olives can be harvested for use as well.

Onion (Allium cepa) a relative of garlic, it has hollow leaves and round underground bulbs. It forms clusters of green-white flowers that appear to be star shaped.

P
Parsley (Petroselinum crispum) a clumpy plant with a white taproot and bright green triangular leaves it is grown in gardens for its fragrance and the look of its tiny yellow-green flowers, as well as served as a garnish or used in recipes. When

eaten in moderation it provides a number of benefits including vitamins A,

C and E and iron, but over use can be toxic.

Passion flower (Passiflora) a fragrant white or lavender flower with 3-5 bright green leaves; it produces yellow fruit that can be eaten raw or cooked. The flowers are used in syrups and when used in combination with other herbs it is a relaxing non-addictive sedative. It has also been used to break drug addiction.

Patchouli (Pogostemon cablin) a bushy evergreen with fragrant velvety leaves, it produces white flowers with violet marks and filaments. It has long been used for its fragrant oil but is instrumental in medicine as well. The leaves can be used for many things from headache and nausea to sexual dysfunction.

Pennyroyal (Mentha pulegium) See mint

Pau d'arco (Tabebuia impetiginosa) a large tree with gray bark and green-gray leaves that are divided into 5-7 leaflets, the tree has a long history of healing such ailments as cancer, stomach ulcers and even rabies. The tree generally flowers pink to purple flowers depending upon species.

Peppermint (Mentha) (*See Mint*)

Plantain (Plantago) a common lawn weed it can be found as a nuisance in most any lawn. Plantain lanceolata or Ribwort can be used interchangeably with plantain major or common plantain. It grows as a flat bunch of broad green leaves with a thin spike of small white flowers growing straight up from its center. Used to treat both internal and external ailment the plants leaves and seeds are also eatable.

Pumpkin (Cucurbita maxima) a trailing or climbing vine with 5 angled stems and broad leaves it blossoms yellow flowers followed by large fruits which may be white, yellow, orange, green, gray or red. The seeds, pulp and fruit may be eaten each used for a different number of ailments

R

Raspberry (Rubus idaeus) see blackberry

Red clover (Trifolium pratense) enriches the soil with nitrogen. It has been used medicinally for menstrual problems as well as cancer. It produces thin stems hat bare a puff of tubular purplish flowers and three leaves that have three leaflets each. The flowers have a sweet taste when suckled which makes it idea for syrups.

Ribwort (Plantago lanceolata) (*See Plantain*)

Rose (Rosa) a family of about 150 different types of roses, they have been used for centuries for their fragrant oils as well as for medicinal purposes. The fruit of the rose, also known as rosehips are high in vitamin C and thus a nutritious snack. They can be eaten raw or made into jellies, candies or syrups.

Rosemary (Rosmarinus officinalis) a fragrant evergreen stalk with many branches and tough blunt ended needles; rosemary is a wonderful addition to gardens as well as kitchens. Some species produce lovely pink, purple, blue or whit flowers that can be added to salads and the whole sprigs can be used in cooking or for medicine.

S

Safflower (Carthamus tinctorius) a thistle like flower that has been used as a coloring agent for centuries, it produces yellow pigments in water and red in alcohol. Also known as false saffron it has tall stems with spiny leaves and yellow thistle like flower heads. It can be used in medicine as well as in cooking to reduce cholesterol levels; it also stimulates the circulation, relieves pain and reduces inflammation.

Saffron (Crocus sativus) used for its flavor and coloring for over 4000 years, saffron has been a prized commodity in gardens and trade. It is noted for its purple blooms but cultivated for its yellow anthers and deep red styles that are divided into 3 branches. It is not to be confused with the meadow saffron that is toxic.

Sage (Salvia) a large group of species that have been used for its beautiful flowers as well as it unique medicinal properties; the sage family includes clary sage, white sage, and common sage to name only a few. Clary sage has remarkable blue, pink or purple flowers on tall stems with light green broad leaves that are slightly hairy. White sage is commonly used in smudging or purification rituals. Common sage is a evergreen shrub with velvety wrinkled leaves and bluish purple flowers.

Sarsaparilla (Aralia nudicaulis) also called wild sarsaparilla is an evergreen shrub that grows in woodland areas. Native Americans used it for the treatment of broken limbs as well as female disorders. It has tiny greenish white flowers that are followed by dark purple berries. Related to the American spikenard, sarsaparilla was the flavoring ingredient in homemade root beer.

Shavegrass (Equisetum arvense) also known as horsetail or bottlebrush it was used in the Middle Ages to scour cookware. They have tall straight stems with spreading branches of green bottle brush like leaves. It is mostly used as an astringent but also act to control internal and external bleeding.

Silverweed (Potentilla anserine) a member of the cinquefoil, it is a slender branched plant whose leaves are covered with a soft downy hair giving it the name silverweed. It has 12-15 pairs of oval leaflet and bright yellow flowers with 5 petals that resemble butter cups. It is used to stop bleeding as well as for cramps and sore throats. It is also useful for skin complaints such as sunburns, pimples and pits due to chicken pox.

Skullcap (Scutellaria lateriflora) also called Virginian skullcap or mad dog skull cap it was once used to treat rabies. It has been used by the Cherokee Indians for menstrual problems and works wonders on moods and tension associated with PMS. It has long thin stems with large jagged leaves and tiny purple, pink, or white flowers that grow in spikes. It has a sedative use and works to aid in withdraw symptoms from drugs.

Slippery elm (Ulmus rubra) a decorative tree it has been widely cultivated for its healing properties. The outer bark has been used to make salves and decoctions for easing childbirth and relieving sore throats, it was once widely used as an abortifacient. The powdered inner bark is still used for some medicinal treatments. It has a fenugreek smell and is made into a gruel that can be flavored with honey and other spices and taken internally for irritable bowel syndrome or other gastric disorders. It can also be used externally for the treatment of wounds.

Soy (Glycine max) a bushy plant with red-gray hairs and trifoliate leaves it has beneficial uses in diet. It resembles estrogen and contains fatty acids that are essential for hormone production. Though not exactly and herb, it has been a staple for a wide range of foods and nutritional uses. It produces small white or pink flowers followed by yellow, brown, gray, or almost black seeds that are used unripened or ripe and fermented.

Squaw vine (Mitchella repens) a mat forming evergreen with shiny white veined leaves; it has been used by Native American tribes to ease childbirth. It has white or pink flowers that are followed by bright red edible berries that relax the uterus and prepares the body for childbirth. It is not used during the first 6 months of pregnancy but may be used during the last 2.

St. John's Wort (Hypericum perforatum) sometimes referred to as natures Prozac due to its claming and mood balancing effect; it was originally used to treat anxiety but is now showing use in treating all sorts of mood disorders including depression. It has long woody stalks with sparse blunt leaves and large yellow flowers with 5 petals which will ooze red when crushed leading to its religious and magical tradition.

Strawberry (Fragaria vesca) a collection of low-growing plants, the strawberry has long been used as a medicinal remedy. The roots and leaves have been used for skin irritations as for stomach upset. The juice is used for the discoloration of teeth and it makes a refreshing treat for hot summer days. It has broad leaves with white 5 petaled flowers that produce bright red berries with the small seed on the skin.

Sundew (Drosera rotundifolia) an ever green insectivourous plant, it was named for the sticky "dew" that forms on the hairy leaflets used to trap bugs and eat them. It has a rosette of long stems that are reddish green and sticky scoop shaped leaves. It bares small white flowers with 5 petals followed by winged seeds.

Sweet marjoram (Origanum majorana) part of the oregano family, it is an evergreen shrub with wiry reddish brown stems and downy green-gray leaves and small white or pink flowers. The flavor is more subtle than that of regular oregano but its uses and properties are similar.

T
Tea tree (Melaleuca alternifolia) related to bottlebrush, this small ever green shrub has papery bark that forms in layers and pointy leaves. It is grown for its small white flowers and used medicinally for fighting fungal, bacterial and viral infections.

Thyme (Thymus) a large collection of small woody based ever greens; thyme has many fragrant species with abundant flowers that produce nectar that is important for bees. The many different types contribute to multiple flavors and uses for seasoning and healing. Thyme can grow on long narrow stalks with various leaf shapes from thin to round and produce a number of colored blooms that can be white, pink, yellow or green. Though usually used for its oils it makes a beautiful addition to gardens and walkways as well.

Tomato (Lycopersicon esculentum) is a vine plant that is related to the potato. It has similar leaves and flowers but produces fruit on the vine instead of underground. It was once thought to be poisonous due to its similarity to henbane, mandrake and deadly nightshade and so linked to witchcraft. Its name is derived from German, which means "edible wolf peach" and was once thought to be connected to werewolves.

V
Valerian (Valeriana officinalis) though for many it smells like old gym socks, valerian is quite attractive to cats. It has been used as a safe sedative that will not react with alcohol. It is a tall clump forming flower with fragrant leaves and small pink or white flowers and tiny hairy seeds. Most commonly the root is used in teas and tinctures the oils are also used for flavors and fragrances. It can also be used to trap rodents and cats who find the aroma irresistible.

W
Watermelon related to the same family as pumpkins cantaloupes and squash, the watermelon is a summer tradition. Its large fruits are grown on long thick vines with subtle flowers that must be pollinated by honey bees in order to produce fruit. The watermelon can vary in size shape and color and may be grow seedless. Contrary to grandma's tale, you will not grow a watermelon plant in your tummy if you swallow the seeds. In fact they are actually good for you. They need to be taken out of the husks or chewed to obtain the nutritional value, or they can be cooked in soups but they are high in zinc and iron. But they

are also high in calories and fat. The typical serving size is one ounce dried seed kernels, but that is a lot for watermelon.

Water mint (Mentha arvensis) See mint.

White Willow (Salix alba) one of many interchangeable types of willow, it is the basis for the pain reliever and anti fever medication aspirin. The willow has grayish bark and long hanging branches with yellow green leaves. It has yellow flowers in the spring and known for its colorful branches in winter. The bark is used in strong teas, powders and decoctions and the leaves are collected and used dried or fresh of infusions.

Wild Yam (Dioscorea villosa) a wild climber with pointed heart shaped leaves, the roots and stems have many medicinal uses including colic in infants and arthritis. The yam is named for the W. African word that means "eat", for its large edible roots. It produces small yellow-green flowers in spikes along it long twining vines.

Witch grass (Agropyron repens) also called couch grass is generally thought of as a common weed. It has been used medicinally since the first century with no known side effects. It is a dull green leaf with stiff spike flowers that grow in a zigzag. It is used to help the kidneys and bowls, lower cholesterol and clear infections.

Witch hazel (Hamamelis virginiana) named for its ties to witchcraft it was used by the Mohawk Indians as a treatment for eyes by steeping the bark in water. This practice was adopted by settlers despite the names association with the occult. The astringent can be found in the first aid section of most stores but is less potent than the tincture made from the plants broad leaves. It has clusters of 2-4 yellow fragrant flowers in the fall that appear as the leaves begin to fall away.

Wood betony (Betonica officinalis) also known as Stachys officinalis, it has been used for medical and magical practices for centuries. Used to cure headaches, it was also regarded to protect and cure the body from witchcraft. It grows on long thick stalks with wrinkled scalloped leaves and tall spikes of deep magenta colored blooms. The leaves and flowers are used to make teas to treat a number of ailments.

Wormwood (Artemisia absinthium) See Mugwort

Y

Yarrow (Achillea millefolium) named for Achilles who supposedly used the herb to heal the wounds of his solders in battle. The flowers are arranged in fragrant clusters each with 5 petals that form a flat top surface. Yarrow is also known as Milfoil. The leaves of the plant are eatable and the blossoms are commonly used in teas.

Yellow dock (Rumex crispus) includes various types of docks and sorrels, this stout root stalk has lance like leaves with wavy margins and tiny green flowers. Used internally and externally for skin conditions too much can cause nausea.

Yerba mate (Ilex paraguariensis) a member of the holly family, it is an ever green tree with pointed oval shaped leaves and small greenish white flowers. The leaves contain caffeine, which makes it ideal for bronchial stimulation or a morning pick me up.

Acknowledgments and references

As I stated at the beginning, I have read a lot of books prior to writing this one. I would like to take the time to acknowledge some of the ones who have been most beneficial to me whether for their inspiration or for their knowledge. It takes a great deal of effort to put together something like this and to all of those who have come before me I have a magnitude of respect. For all who come after me, best of luck and my deepest sympathies to you. It has been quiet a trial but still satisfying to put this together. I certainly hope the readers find it useful.

For the inspiration:

The Herbal Drug Store; Linda B. White MD, Steven Foster and the staff of Herbs for   Health,   copy   write 2000 by Rondale Inc.

Cunningham's   Encyclopedia   of   Magical   Herbs; Scott Cunningham, copy write 1984 by   L l e w w l l y n ' s publications St. Paul, Minnesota

The Herb Society of America New Encyclopedia of Herbs and Their Uses; Deni Bown,   copy write 2001 by DK Publishing New York, NY

Online sites that have been helpful:

Botanica.com
Wiccanwisdom.tripod.com
Sagemountain.com
Wildroots.com
Moonsmuse.com
Mymagicshop.com
Trilightherbs.com
Liferesearchuniversal.com

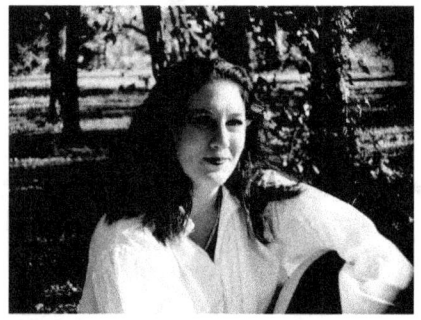

P.M. Schamel lives in Oklahoma with her husband and son as well as the family dog, 2 cats, 1 rat and various rescued strays that pop in from time to time. She enjoys tending her own herb, flower and vegetable gardens and shares with her husband the responsibility of hunting for the family. Her joys of gardening and natural gifts in magical healing were the inspiration for this book.